APPLIED THEATRE IN PAEDIATRICS

This book explores applied theatre practice for children in environments of illness and cure and how it can powerfully normalise children's hospitalisation experience. It is an essential tool for making meaning of children's illness, putting it into a fictional context and developing better control of their clinical experiences. It can be central to raising the standards of care and quality of life during illness.

Taken from the author's research and participatory bedside theatre practice in hospitals before, during and after the COVID-19 pandemic, this book demonstrates new learning about aesthetics, ethics, emotions, stories, puppetry, digital arts and research methodologies about children's health and wellbeing. It provides a selection of ten unique stories told by children inspired by applied theatre practice in paediatrics, cardiac, oncology, neurosurgery, burns units and complex and intensive care wards. Stories aid in understanding the language of children's pain for a better assessment and management of pain by healthcare professionals through the arts. It analyses synergistic theatre performance in 'stitched lands' between challenging realities and safe fictionalities. This book enables artists to develop new ways of thinking and contributes to further improvements in the provision of education and reflective learning in the field.

It also addresses the emotional labour of the artist in healthcare and makes recommendations for balanced training to prevent emotional exhaustion.

Designed for artists, healthcare professionals, therapists, play specialists and teachers who work with children in healthcare, this text aims to help many people find creative ways of making a positive difference in sick children's lives. It is a book for those who love and care for children.

Persephone Sextou is a professor in applied theatre for health and wellbeing and the director of the Sidney De Haan Research Centre at Canterbury Christ Church University. She is a leading expert in participatory dramas for sick children in hospitals with 30 years of experience in academia around the world. She is the proud mother of two and the author of *Theatre for Children in Hospital: The Gift of Compassion*.

Learning through Theatre: Dramatic Opportunities, Engagements and Challenges
Series Editors
John O'Toole and Kelly Freebody

This series commissions in-depth studies of the use of theatre and drama for the widest range of specific purposes – beyond entertainment itself – that involve learning. Contexts include formal educational settings such as schools and colleges, as well as social, communal, health, political, developing world, human services, war zones and commercial contexts. In the fields of applied theatre and drama education, three paradigms often define the purpose and the practice:

- drama as *art*
- drama as *education*
- drama as social action and change.

Books in the series tackle both the opportunities and the tensions among these paradigms: the developments, the challenges and the achievements in this still-growing field. Critical awareness and appraisal are a key feature, with some titles primarily grounded in theory and analysis, some more illustrative of good and bad practice. Authors include pioneers and established leaders as well as emerging practitioners and scholars.

Teaching and Learning Through Dramaturgy: Education as an Artful Engagement
Anna-Lena Østern

Applied Theatre in Paediatrics
Stories, Children and Synergies of Emotions
Persephone Sextou

For more information, please visit: https://www.routledge.com/Learning-Through-Theatre/book-series/LTT

APPLIED THEATRE IN PAEDIATRICS

Stories, Children and Synergies of Emotions

Persephone Sextou

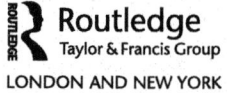

LONDON AND NEW YORK

Designed cover image: Persephone Sextou

First published 2023
by Routledge
4 Park Square, Milton Park, Abingdon, Oxon OX14 4RN

and by Routledge
605 Third Avenue, New York, NY 10158

Routledge is an imprint of the Taylor & Francis Group, an informa business

© 2023 Persephone Sextou

The right of Persephone Sextou to be identified as author of this work has been asserted in accordance with sections 77 and 78 of the Copyright, Designs and Patents Act 1988.

All rights reserved. No part of this book may be reprinted or reproduced or utilised in any form or by any electronic, mechanical, or other means, now known or hereafter invented, including photocopying and recording, or in any information storage or retrieval system, without permission in writing from the publishers.

Trademark notice: Product or corporate names may be trademarks or registered trademarks, and are used only for identification and explanation without intent to infringe.

British Library Cataloguing-in-Publication Data
A catalogue record for this book is available from the British Library

ISBN: 978-0-367-48325-8 (hbk)
ISBN: 978-0-367-48326-5 (pbk)
ISBN: 978-1-003-03934-1 (ebk)

DOI: 10.4324/9781003039341

Typeset in Bembo
by Apex CoVantage, LLC

*To my husband Michalis and my children Eleni and Nektarios,
who make my world worth living.*

CONTENTS

Preface ix
Acknowledgements xiv

1 Hospitalised children's stories in applied theatre 1
  A synergistic and eudemonic phenomenon 1
  Stories in-betweenness 6
  Communicating pain: a process of attunement 9
  Applied theatre or play therapy? 11
  The 'fictional bubble': explosions and interruptions 14
  The act of caring 15
  The 'marginal participant' technique 16

2 Applied theatre and digital assets on the wards 21
  The 'Rocket-Arts' project in hospitals 21
    Pre-pandemic bedside performance 23
    Post-pandemic digital solutions 25
    Collection of stories 26
    The impact of COVID-19 on 'Rocket-Arts' 29

3 Sick children's stories: from patients to story-makers 31
  Introduction to stories 31
  Jane: 'The piano is on fire' 33
  Sheila: 'A moon made of cheese' 35
  Paul: 'The naughty Wolf' 37
  Alex: 'My grandfather's wellies' 39

Sandy: 'We need the Pancakes' 42
Claire: 'Silence' 43
Karim: 'No!' 45
Lisa: 'A robot who could not dance' 46
Melissa: 'The Planetary' 47
Margaret: 'A park for the animals' 49
   Stories of hospitalisation on a stitched land 52

4   Applied performance, puppetry and hospital tuition   60
The 'Bird Island' project 60
Lollie the rough collie and the magic kiss 61
Feeling worried in paediatrics 62
The dramatic frame 63
Participatory puppetry in hospital 64
Research 66
Complementing artistic knowing 68
Emma's story 72
Katarina's story 73
Azeeb's story 74

5   Caring enough is never enough: training actors on
    emotional skills   78
Reflective poetry in paediatrics 78
   Reflections 80
Walking the labyrinth on the ward: a metaphor 84
Caring for the artist: we can't pour from an empty cup! 85
Emotional awareness: an act of caring 87
Realisations to take forward 90
Who is the excellent actor in healthcare? A portrait 92

6   The future: questions and recommendations   97
A flashback: my practice in a nutshell 97
Post-pandemic learning 101
Time for change 108
   Actions by healthcare providers 110
   Actions by local authorities and governments 111
   Actions by artists 111

Appendix A Rocket-Arts' or Simba, the therapy dog. The script   115
Appendix B 'Lollie the rough collie and the magic kiss'. The story   120
Index   123

PREFACE

This book is for those who love and care for children, their emotions and their stories as powerful experiences of joyful moments in illness. Every child's story is entirely individual. Every child sees life through their filters. Every reading has its powers. Those who care for sick children tend to their imaginative stories. Can stories offer children control over their emotions and experience of illness? Can making stories help them play with the images and experiences they have and gain a clearer understanding of how life is, a better vision of who they are, how they feel, who they want to become, what path they want to walk and what steps to change they should take creatively? Children may tell stories to escape from reality, to attract our attention and ask for help.

Stories make us human. We tell stories to make sense of what we experience in life and connect with others in good and bad times. We review and revise the past through our stories, understand and tolerate the present and visualise tomorrow. We use stories to travel in time. We tell stories to reach out for the imagined and the possible. Stories are ways of demystifying the mystery of life, revealing hidden truths and emotions. Stories of birth. Stories of love. Stories of pain. Stories of illness. Stories of hope. Stories of death. Stories of escape. Stories of regret. Stories of forgiveness. Stories of growth. We share our emotions with people we know well, those we trust, people we have just met, and others we hope to meet and unite through our stories.

I have been working with children in various roles since 1992, and I can confirm from my experience that children are masters of imagination. They have a unique gift, a capacity to pull threads from their worlds and use them in stories that can create connections between them and their characters, between their own experiences and the experiences of others. In addition, they do not even care about how adults will perceive their stories. Most children's stories are genuine, original and spontaneous. They come from an authentic place, and thus, they may sound bold, dramatic, cruel, direct and resentful. Yet it is through listening to what children say in their stories that we have an opportunity to engage with the craft of truthful and brave storytelling, as only children know. Using our intuition, we can sense the meaning behind the children's words, the magnificence of joy behind the moment of sharing and the learning behind the pain. So many old and new story forms, themes, archetypical myths, tales and images offer us an insight into cultures and traditions. So many inspirations, journeys and destinations take us to imagined worlds. And yet, children make stories with no use of guidelines, no pattern, structure or scaffolding theories, and any desire to make meaning to others or affect people's lives in any possible way. Each child is unique, and so are their stories.

By seeing with the eyes of our souls, we can see children's worlds more rightly and empathetically to gain a stronger sense of understanding children and their emotions in times of illness. I do not seek to analyse or explain the delight and reward of hearing a story from a child in paediatrics. The pleasure and reward need no explaining. However, my continuous learning from working with children in hospitals for over 20 years has drawn my attention to a persistent need to discuss the role of stories that sick, injured and terminally ill children tell in applied theatre contexts. I have found that some children who experience illness and pain tend to devise stories about sickness and pain, fear and loss. The difference is that pain, anxiety and loss are experiences that happen to others in their stories. It occurs to family animals and heroes they know from picture books; it happens to familiar toys. It happens to everyday insignificant objects that become significant in moments of loneliness and silence.

Over the years, I realised that bedside theatre performance creates a particular openness. There is no one culture here, no single idea, no expectation of what the children should do; so if the actors tell children that a story is a heaven of opportunity, kindness, possibility and escape to imagined worlds, a place where everyone is invited to be who they wish to be and say what they feel is the right thing to say or remain silent, then, actually, children believe them. In my projects in paediatrics, actors have conspired to tell children that magical boots can fly to the moon, dragons can have ears made of eggplants and a glittering star can be touched. It is the child's right to own the potential of stories; how to create them, live them, change them, remake them, neglect them, revive them and perform them with assistance, when needed, from actors. So that is one reason why the stories of this book are so good: the actors who worked with hospitalised children expect and believe that they can be playful and creative in illness, and as a researcher, I support this creation.

Something magical happens when we tell children stories about accepting that it is normal to be sick. Amazingly, the fear of illness melts away for a while when the children are liberated from their role as patients and become creative participants in storytelling performances. Storytelling becomes a listening experience, a process for thinking, evaluating and understanding (Wilson 2022). I have seen hospitalised children becoming engaged in the dramatic conditions of space and time and escaping their scary realities through fiction. By researching children's spontaneous reactions to bedside performance in hospitals, I discovered that the children's continuous immersion in fictional situations is a 'strategy' that many children follow subconsciously to improve their ability to deal with real problems that they experience because of illness and hospitalisation. Storytelling in participatory bedside theatre strengthens and refines the paths that lead to competent navigation of life's experiences during illness. In theatre, problems can be remedied by enacting the imagined experience (story). Through theatre, children can 'ease' the emotional experience of being with illness because it brings it closer to the audience's attention in ordinary situations that people can relate to. For theatre and stories to do this, I wrote this book to continue my discussions about stories and emotions and explore the synergy of applied theatre practice that involves storytelling, puppetry, toy theatre and toy-based films in environments of illness more closely. However, emotions and illness can be complex, taboo issues that people are hesitant to openly discuss for fear of upsetting others or becoming upset by talking about them. And yet, there is a need to use cases of stories in paediatrics as a paradigm to acknowledge the importance of remembering that a happy childhood is a ticket to happy adult life.

The children as story-makers represented here all spent time at various hospitals in Birmingham, West Midlands in England. Birmingham is a multi-cultural city of three million people, a cultural blend of histories and languages worldwide. Some of the children who participated in my projects came to English or at least wrote English after five or six years. That was either because of developmental delays, health conditions, learning disabilities or difficulties, or migration. Therefore, a 'locked-in' period in their lives may have been challenging because communication was restricted and isolation was painful. However, I think that, as with all things in life, there may have been a time for those children to stay with their silent and develop their voices. It may also account for the personal treasures, the thoughts and the hidden emotions of so many of their stories. The stories of this book are charged with emotions because they came from the children's hearts, and for all the sadness they may record, they are joyous and humorous because they are about finding a glimpse of happiness in difficulty. Therefore, they are expected to affect the readers' hearts too.

Exploring the potential for applied theatre as a creative practice for health and wellbeing encounters a need to reconsider the art form's power in shaping the language of aesthetics in healthcare contexts and restoring agency to patients in partnership with healthcare professionals. I could have chosen to describe several bedside performances to illustrate arguments within applied theatre in paediatrics. However, I decided to focus on the stories, the dialogues, words spoken and implied, the emotions, the reactions and interactions during the performance as I witnessed them from my perspective and practical experience. I make no apologies that the examples of my seeing do not aim to offer a critique of the problematic integration of applied arts in healthcare. This is not the scope of this book, as most of it is covered in my previous writings. Applied theatre in paediatrics should pay attention to the methods of the process and the relationships between actors and patients as participants, not the specifics of the hospital sites and policies. The above is disclaimed as an apology for the inevitable overstepping of clinicians' and therapists' boundaries in the analysis of practices, stories and moments that I have witnessed by a non-expert in healthcare and therapeutic professions. I am not a psychologist, therapist or emotions analyst but an applied theatre researcher meeting these specialities at certain moments in clinical settings. I use critical reflections of my practice as a researcher in paediatrics as a paradigm, a way of looking at exchanges of emotions between actors and children. However, my research aims to appeal to a broader audience of actors in paediatrics, such as community actors, puppeteers, health play specialists and creative therapists, because it addresses shared concerns and challenges. The idea is that the actor in paediatrics is an example of an artist in healthcare, a studied and evaluated case of performing in social settings. This contrasts with the idea that the actor who works with children in hospitals is an undeveloped and remote example of artistic practice. Hence, my experience in children's hospitals applies to the broader context of contemporary and cross-disciplinary applied theatre and participatory arts practice with vulnerable audiences and communities. This book reflects my applied theatre model in paediatrics, its practice and the challenges emerging from entering a clinical culture as an actor, and my reflections on examples of process-based and participatory projects with children bedside. The chapters build on my research and delve deeper into exploring applied theatre for children in difficult circumstances because of illness and their emotional experience in interactive performance.

It may be hard to hear the stories from the theatre in paediatrics without reflecting on one's practice and personal life. For me, theatre for children in hospitals has been more than the arts-based, knowledge-transfer research I conduct, the way I return something to the community, a form of artistic and political intervention. The children's stories help me understand fear, pain, courage and bravery in my own life. Applied theatre in paediatrics has become a path to becoming a more conscious, compassionate person. My book '*Theatre for children in hospital*' (Sextou 2016) is a chronicle of that journey. It revealed the importance of accepting theatre as a way of adding a playful dimension to sick children's lives with sensitivity, respect, love, empathy and compassion. I offered explicit instructions for making and evaluating imaginative theatre projects for children in hospitals that appeal to experienced practitioners and newcomers interested in using theatre to entertain, relax and help children and their families maintain their optimism about life in hospitals and during recovery. The present book is aimed to become a vehicle for bringing some of the stories actors told to children and some of the hospitalised children's stories to a larger audience of readers. The reader will see how stories add to the notion of what it means to be a child with ill health and hopefully gain an insight into how we can support sick children better. I hope that by reading the stories of children who are often worried, the professionals who work with them will improve their understanding of children as patients and find the strength to actively listen to the children's needs. I hope that children whose experience of illness was somewhat invisible to nurses, doctors, parents and families will become more visible, heard and widely respected. Finally, I hope those stories will enable us to think again about survival, patience, joy, gratefulness and possibility.

References

Sextou, P 2016, *Theatre for Children in Hospital. The Gift of Compassion*, Intellect: Bristol.
Wilson, M 2022, *Storytelling: (Arts for Health)*, Emerald Publishing Limited: London.

Bibliography

Armstrong, K 2005, *A Short History of Myth*, Canongate Books: Edinburg.
Boyd, B 2009, *On the Origin of Stories. Evolution, Cognition and Fiction*, The Belknap Press of Harvard University: Cambridge, MA.

ACKNOWLEDGEMENTS

Let us acknowledge the difficulties hospitalised children and their families go through when reading and thinking about them in this book.

Let us hold in mind those children who have spent days, weeks, months and years in hospital and palliative care, and all those who have died in hospitals around the world.

Let us think of pain as one of the most difficult aspects of life, given that pain is subjective, private experience and personal.

Let us appreciate that stories use metaphorical language as a resource in understanding and communicating emotions to others.

Let us embrace the challenge of performing at sick and injured children's bedsides, and all those actors who have been brave to exchange emotions with audiences through the art form.

Let us be self-aware about our thoughts, reflections and interpretations of the stories as products of participation and sharing.

Let us be gentle with ourselves and others in this challenging territory of fiction that is incubated within what can be a daunting reality.

1
HOSPITALISED CHILDREN'S STORIES IN APPLIED THEATRE

I am delighted to bring this chapter to readers as an opener and hope that it will stimulate their interest and that the range of concepts offered here will be helpful to the related chapters I discuss. Aiming to contextualise applied theatre in paediatrics, I discuss the synergistic nature and beauty of audience participation in bedside performance to argue that the exchange of strength or weakness, power or vulnerability, control or obedience relates to the actor–child relationship. I will discuss how stories between reality and fictionality provide a safe and positive environment for a reassuring experience. I am interested in the concept of 'attunement', the actor's reactiveness to the child-patient as a participant in performance rather than as a patient. Therefore, I will try to demystify the bias and wrong assumptions of the many that theatre in hospital is aimed to heal. I will define the nature of theatre audiences in paediatrics and the importance of evaluating applied theatre practice in hospitals as an act of caring for these audiences. Finally, I will explain how using the 'marginal participant technique' creates opportunities for an objective distancing to witness the dramatic action in paediatrics.

A synergistic and eudemonic phenomenon

Applied theatre in paediatrics is a synergistic phenomenon. Since I was studying ancient Greek at school, I have always liked the etymology of the word synergy from the Greek (ΣΥΝΕΡΓΕΙΑ). ΣΥΝ 'together' and ΕΡΓΟΝ 'work' have the same root that gives us energy (ΕΝΕΡΓΕΙΑ). Ergon is a unit of energy. When one work magnifies the effect of another, together, they have synergy. When ingredients are combined, it is often expected that these will interact differently in chemistry. When something unexpected happens, this is *synergy* or 'magic'. In human interaction, incredible things happen when combinations of elements interact. For example, when people work together, they bring their energy resources to create

DOI: 10.4324/9781003039341-1

something greater than they could do alone. That more extraordinary achievement can be called 'magic'. In applied theatre in paediatrics, performance is a synergistic cooperative action. The actor and the child combine their energies, voices, narratives, moods, emotions, skills and references to create collaborative stories in a complementary role. From my long experience in this discipline, I recall that extra sparkle in children's eyes when their faces are lit up in performance. I remember that unique moment of connection between the child and the actor when they use an object creatively. I recall that sense of achievement and joy when the child decides how the story should end. All these moments can be 'magic' too. Synergy in bedside performance can be remarkable not only because it takes place under challenging circumstances defined by ill health but also because it demonstrates if nothing else can, that the unexpected creative outcome and the possible remains during illness.

The value implicit in synergistic performance is essential for practitioners and audiences with whom they work. In the dramatic situation, the exchange of strength or weakness, power or vulnerability, control or obedience relates to the actor–child relationship. I believe that it is not only the content of the stories that are affected by synergies but also how the stories are told and retold in paediatrics. How stories are created with vulnerable individuals and communities raises ethical concerns about the practice, especially about the invitation to participation (Thompson 2005). Actors often argue that they act within fiction that protects the audience and themselves from their emotional exchanges when interacting. However, I am aware that some performances may become a joined product of synergistic activity where the personalities of the artist and the child influence the outcome. Some stories may reveal children's feelings and moods through metaphors and parables. Still, there is always a caution that there is uncertainty about whether those feelings are genuine or have been affected by the interaction with the actor. It is possible that the personal feelings of the actor can intrude into the dialogues with the child during the participatory performance. While working with children in hospital wards, I realised that stories we tell and stories that the children create become inevitably tools through which children connect and communicate with actors. Connection occurs 'in-imagination' during the fictional conditions of space and time. This demonstrates that participatory theatre practice in hospitals has origins and consequences for actors and children. It also raises complex ethical research questions about the authorship and ownership of the stories. There is a question, for example, of how these stories as products of co-creation and synergy between the actor and the child become stories of one teller and who the teller is. The boundaries of authorship, ownership and responsibility become indistinct because actors and vulnerable children are involved in the performance as participants.

Howell et al. (2015) discuss the concept of 'fuzzy boundaries' in a visual research context. Fuzzy boundaries relate to the confusion of roles between researchers and participants in the research process, which involves vulnerable people. They argue that blurred boundaries lead to the development of intense feelings of responsibility towards the research participant, which may impact the researchers' view of the purposes and outcomes of the research project. I feel a great responsibility towards the children who participated in bedside dramas and the actors who engaged children in interactive experiences through drama. I am constantly aware of the need to employ an ethical approach to applied theatre in hospitals by reflecting on the implications of bedside theatre practice. While acknowledging the moral dimensions of research with hospitalised children, blurred boundaries are a potential research issue involving the co-creation of stories with vulnerable people. The actors probably consider that they have an inclusive and democratic approach to hospitalised children as participants in the performance. However, to be realistic, sometimes inclusive and democratic may be superficial. We can also make sympathetic noises about participatory ownership of the performance, breaking down the barriers between audiences and actors in the hospital as long as the actors control the implementation. It may be that the innovative and pioneering nature of the work results in such questions about ownership and authorship with the potential to challenge accepted conventional approaches to arts-based research. However, it also allows for an acceptance of renovating sick children's identities from patients to creative story-makers.

Of course, there is an excellent opportunity for discussing participation regarding inspiration, identity and ownership of the stories. The reader is encouraged to think of the stories as products of a dialogue between the child and the actor and between the child and the world. Sakr et al. (2015) argue that by exploring arts-making ideas with children, we can better understand children's internal 'self' in a dialogue with the external world. In my practice, a unique type of audience participation during an open-ending, flexible performance is defined by inter-play. Starting from the notion that children who are ill still want to and providing sick children with play opportunities may improve the quality of their health play (Lindon 2002), I problematise hospitals as sites of opportunity for playful synergies and making of stories. I will present some of these stories in Chapter 3. These are stories of creativity, hope, inspiration and unwavering courage. I will discuss in what sense applied theatre inspires children to open up and reveal their feelings and how active participation in performance enhances a shift of identity from 'I am ill and I cannot play' to 'I am ill and I can play', and how stories enact children's experience of illness. How do creative practices work to alter our preconceptions about identities of illness, abilities and powers? How does the art form enable synergies between the actor and the child, and how might those synergies illuminate important ideas or develop creative processes and engagement with learning?

I admit that I am dubious about the meaning of learning and the claim of knowing in this area of research. We live in a society where value is placed on understanding, learning, measuring and considering facts, aiming, achieving and being sure about research outcomes. However, we often do not know, we cannot understand and we are unable to see clearly and guarantee conclusions over facts. Sometimes in theatre, as in life, not knowing is OK. Sepinuck (2013), in her book '*Theatre of Witness*', gives voice to marginalised people whose stories have been untold or unlisted, creating a safe environment for them to learn without judgment through theatre. She argues that not knowing allows us to explore further, see deeper, listen more actively, and want to experience and feel more with little expectation of the outcome. It means that the actor meets people willing to trust that their stories will reveal what needs to be known by trusting the creative process. 'It is fine to wait, to listen, just to let oneself be in the "not knowing". Not knowing is a state of open receptivity' (Sepinuck 2013, p. 227). One of the puzzles that my work often addresses is not applied theatre's purpose in paediatrics but applied theatre's 'centrality' to the overall experience of 'not knowing'. What we don't know with our minds does not rule what we know with our hearts. A dictum from the Pensées (1669) by Blaise Pascal says, 'The heart has its reasons, which reason does not know'. Antoine de Saint-Exupéry (1943) wrote in his novella 'The Little Prince' 'It is only with the heart that one can see rightly, what is essential is invisible to the eye'. That was the Little Prince's secret of knowing in other ways. He learned to invest time, care and effort to connect with a rose and a fox, feeling responsible for them, which made him happy. Because of that empathic connection, the Little Prince saw the importance of caring, listening to, supporting and belonging to someone. I find this story filled with unique opportunities for eudemonic experiences relevant to participating in theatre in paediatrics.

My philosophy about using the arts in healthcare is rooted in Aristotle's theory of wellbeing and happiness, known as 'eudaimonia', the demon of good actions. In Aristotle's eudemonic model of wellbeing, goodness is recognised as a process and outcome of kindness, respect, and sharing knowledge and experience with others in constant interaction with the environment. According to Gallagher et al. (2009), eudaimonia grows from one's well-intended activities that produce good results for the community and the society. Eudaimonia embraces elements of discovery into how individuals can reach their potential in their private lives and interaction with others. I introduced the concept of eudaimonia in my applied theatre practice in hospitals some years ago (Sextou 2016) to argue that eudaimonia is an exceptional quality of happiness, a much more advanced sense of satisfaction that can be earned from creating experiences through theatre with a caring, empathetic and compassionate interest for the ill children. That makes a life worth living.

Applied theatre presents opportunities for eudaimonia by engaging with hospitalised children in intimate performances and integrating the arts further into healthcare systems. By 'integrating', I mean to make the arts more than 'Aw! That would be nice to offer to sick children'. It would mean making bedside theatre, alongside other participatory arts, a mainstream healthcare service and making participation in arts more available to children in hospitals. It would mean making it possible for the actor to improve their capacity to understand children's worlds and their truth of experience better. It would also mean defining the child as an audience, a participant in creativity, rather than an ill person, a patient. Recognising the child as a valued participant enables a synergistic and democratic relationship between the actor and the child where both the actor and the child have a voice, access and ownership of the stories they hear and make. To me, the secret of eudemonic activity lies within the interaction between children and actors in which sick and injured children are recognised as participants and co-creators in the arts rather than participants in illness.

Over the years, I realised that applied theatre practice could incorporate participatory activities such as performance, drama, storytelling, puppetry and toy theatre for children's health and wellbeing. Hospitalised children participating in arts-based activities can be healthier, happier and more resilient in coping with stressful hospital experiences (Lopez-Bushnell & Berg 2018). I use a diverse range of participatory activities in my practice to create paths of communication and experiences of being together in the moment with joy and compassion and to help actors and children connect and develop relationships through a collective process. Participatory arts-based activities found that they distract hospitalised children's minds from the pain and positively impact stress reduction and psychological and physiological wellbeing (Eisen 2006; Sextou 2016; Astles 2020). Witnessing those moments of creative distraction, connection and stress reduction has been a rewarding, even eudemonic experience for me. Through the arts in healthcare, the actor learns to invite children into the centre of their world with kindness. The actor aims to create opportunities for making meaning of what it feels to be a child in illness and what can be done to improve children's lives through the arts concerning their circumstances. When the child and the actor get involved in synergistic bedside performance, they connect, share stories and emotions, and play within the fictional conditions of the arts as witnesses of a eudemonic phenomenon. They are not alone anymore at times of struggle. Nevertheless, there remains a persistent gap in knowledge and analysis around the deeper meanings and functions of emotions' influence on actors and audiences in less ordinary theatrical settings, which rise to unpredictable incidents.

The choice of writing a book to address the eudemonic synergies between actors and children in telling stories together in medical settings is not arbitrary but intentional. The book takes care to support the actor in supporting vulnerable children. It aims to contribute to further improvements in the provision of education and reflective learning in applied theatre as a multi-purpose and cross-disciplinary practice beyond entertainment. Benefits for children in the hospital include body and mind relaxation, a distraction from illness and pain, improvement in behaviours towards taking medication, creative interaction with actors, improved communication with clinical professionals and enhanced social wellbeing (Sextou & Hall 2015). However, the need is not to accurately capture children's emotions in a book about applied theatre but to respond to the oppressiveness of contemporary cultures that either hide or ignore feelings because feelings disappear in silence and social isolation. For the first time, a book deals in-depth with an aspect of applied theatre for children in hospitals that speaks to actors' fears, prejudices and insights about the emotional experience in clinical settings. It draws on the importance of telling bedside stories within intimate hospital performance. It critically explores alternative ways of telling stories in hospitals in times of isolation and loneliness during the pandemic lockdowns. Eudaimonia is particularly well suited to the use of theatre practice for expressing emotions in response to loneliness and despair. Or, simply, it can allow recognition that performing for children in paediatrics is exceptional communication directly revealing the nature of the human heart and its desire to connect and interact with others through stories.

Stories in-betweenness

In the context of paediatrics, stories are products of a dramatic process that flourishes in conditions between two worlds, the world of reality (hospital) and the world of fiction. In drama, as much as in children's play, participants live in the real and fictional worlds. O'Toole (1992, p. 26) describes entering a dramatic situation as 'entering a "play-frame" that provides some protection from external consequences for those who step inside it'. In participatory performance in hospitals, the dramatic story is presented 'as if' it is real. This is where learning occurs, between 'territory' or *metaxis*. Augusto Boal described *metaxis* as the belonging of the participant to two different and autonomous worlds simultaneously: the fictional, the image of reality and the objective reality of the image.

> In any theatre performance, there is likely to be . . . an element of aesthetic distance which enables the audience both to believe and not to believe at the same time. We can imaginatively embrace the fictional world and be caught up in the excitement, fantasy, dangers, and dilemmas it may generate, but we are equally conscious of its fictionality. Boal has described this rather extraordinary paradox as metaxis.
>
> *(Boal 1995, p. 43)*

Metaxis describes the condition of 'in-betweenness' as the state of being placed between others, one of the qualities of being human. The stories of this book are products of using the opportunities created for the audience to be placed between real, being in the hospital, and non-real, being in a spacecraft. In that position, children are invited to express their ideas and feelings and develop a sense of humour and playfulness. The stories are by-products of a dialogue between what is real and what is believed *as if* it was real. The real world is marked by illness. A child might think, 'I am an ill person'. The fictional world is created with imagination. It allows the child to rethink their role 'I am an astronaut travelling to Mars'. This is 'empathetic engagement' and is enabled by the dramatic context and the conditions of safety it generates. It is safe for one to be the 'other' person and act like someone else without facing the consequences of their decisions and actions, as in real life. Children and actors meet on the metaphorical ground within an aesthetic framework and the dramatic conditions of space, time, focus and tension (Jackson 2007). Within the protection of the metaphorical ground (e.g. on an adventure in space), children may imaginatively recreate the hospital experience in their own words and bring life and form to the most common issues pertinent to children in illness. In the stories, it is expected that one can admire children's capacity to describe and express aspects of their experiences, both reflectively and creatively. This may be conscious or unconscious and relates to the relationship between real and fictional contexts.

John O'Toole (1992, p. 234) argues that 'the metaxis between the real and the fictional contexts always exists where there is powerful drama'. Within the drama, the fictional context is negotiable and flexible, offering the participants relaxed conditions where they can take the fictional context seriously or not, where they have the liberty to accept, reject or alter the drama conditions. Children's ability to engage with the imaginary situation and commit to drama and the actor's ability to frame the problem in drama and set up the conventions are essential to establishing the fictional context. Why is this so important to hospital theatre? The clinical environment as a real context is dominant and cannot be changed or undermined. If actors enter the real context without framing their role in the drama as actors, the child may believe them as real and feel cheated, which is ethically wrong. The actor must employ drama to define what is real and what is not and allow responses between the two. O'Toole continues with permission granted by the fiction, the fictional may allow reality to be suspended, but the real context remains. In the betweenness of fantasy and truth, tensions and resolutions take place. However, a less direct approach is how children respond to fiction and reality in hospitals. Stories enhance children's creativity by offering opportunities to visualise places and characters beyond what is real (the here and now in the hospital) to use their imagination as a ticket to a transformed reality. This means that stories children tell welcome what seems to be their way of transforming their existence in their imagination by 'seeing' themselves in a fictional place and time within the dramatic conventions of theatre. In this way, perhaps children gain control over their circumstances by 'escaping' to a different reality, their fantasyland. We must not forget that some parts or all of some stories are fiction, including invented elements and products of children's imagination, and other stories capture, replicate and immerse experiences from both worlds.

Imagination enables and maintains *metaxis*. This can be serious fun. As children enter the fantasyland in their pretend play, they confront monsters, heroes, spaceships and unicorns. Gottschall (2012) argues that we all humans, children included, are storytelling animals who make up stories to act out our problems and trouble. 'Sometimes the trouble is routine, . . . But often, trouble is existential' (Gottschall 2012, p. 33). We might want to consider what can be discovered about 'what is at stake' within stories. Fictional stories, like play, allow humans to take emotional risks and use emotional resources needed to be in difficulty without exposing themselves to actual risk (Boyd 2009). The images, selected memories and experiences in the stories children tell in paediatrics may represent the 'truth' or what is believed 'as if it's the truth'. However, they may also be pure products of the imagination that could easily mislead the reader. I witnessed the power of children's imagination using true-to-life images and experiences selectively during their stay in the hospital. Once these are triggered by a hospital incident such as hearing someone crying in the next bed or a sensation such as needle pain, children blend them with fiction, adding more drama to the story as it happens in the theatre. Imagination and memory have the power to work well together. One feeds the other, especially in more generally creative writing activities and the arts. The images and words in children's stories may have meaning to the children who used them, a sense that may be unique to them and very different from my world of memories and experiences. We need ways to 'read' these stories with respect and awareness of the risk of making interpretations. When you read the stories in Chapter 3, ask yourself for a glimpse of doubt. And yet, we need ways of getting into the realm of children's imagination and getting out of the rational adult way of thinking. We may better capture how children feel and appreciate their genuine storytelling skills without judgment.

If we suppose that the physical space in a hospital is meant for clinical purposes, then metaxis not only symbolises the use of bedside space in drama but also establishes in-betweenness as the state of placing performance between the clinical and the metaphorical conditions. The area in the hospital occupied by the audience and the actors during the performance and characterised by the theatrical relationship fostered between the two is different from the dramatic space as we know it in the theatre. The 'theatrical space' in the hospital is a private space for the child in a specific site of identity and semiotics. Placing the actor too close to a child's bedside may make feel uncomfortable with them so close, invading the child's emotional space. The desire to transform confined spaces in clinical settings into theatrical spaces can be challenging for that reason. In this sense, applied theatre in paediatrics is classified as site-specific because it is designed for a particular location. If removed from that location, it loses its purpose and meaning. The space and the place are negotiated as the audience's perception of the 'site' is not fixed but open to personal understandings (Birch & Tompkins 2012). Between the children's beds and a chair, the actor uses a range of media to symbolise the space where the story takes place and create warm and colourful imagined worlds within the existent cold hospital environment. In my practice, actors may be restricted by space and technical equipment around children's beds, and therefore, they do not create sets for performances. But, they use puppets as small as a finger and as big as a real-life five-year-old child, as well as other props. They use miniature objects and toys designed to fit in shoe boxes and tiny bags, the minimum of costume-just a pair of glasses, rainbow hats with long silk ribbons attached, shawls, all small things that can symbolise different characters in the drama, portable trees with fairy lights where birds and butterflies live and space rockets standing on clinical drips. The use of space is particularly significant for performing in clinical environments because it disturbs the norm of what a hospital should look like and changes the site's function from an environment for treatment (real world) to a space with artistic potential (imagined world).

For the actor, this transformation requires an awareness of the dynamics between the site's purpose and the theatre's intention to enable the change to develop. That explains why applied theatre in paediatrics represents an ambitious and revolutionary re-interpretation of theatre and hospital. Actors enter the clinical space as out-comers, outsiders, visitors and guests (Thompson 2012), ideally, not as intruders. Guests often visit new places that are different from what they know from experience, with ignorance and naivety. Ignorance as a term to describe the lack of knowledge and awareness of healthcare systems and the processes followed by clinical staff is not necessarily bad. In truth, the actor's ignorance in this context can also benefit them by creating the desire to know more, explore more and achieve more. For example, ignorance opens the opportunity to seek knowledge and make discoveries by asking new questions about space usage in a hospital without a theatre stage. Questions about the dimensional restrictions of the confined space next to a hospital bed can lead to creative solutions by using, for instance, a miniature theatre stage. Actors still have a choice to transform the real (clinical) space into an imagined 'reality' or let the clinical space dominate the artistic experience through what most actors call 'vibes of illness' in a healthcare setting. This book presents stories created within these vibes of illness around sick children's beds. Hopefully, in a small way, I will illustrate the vital role applied theatre practice has as a vehicle of expression for the child in healthcare and the potential of transforming the physical space into a story-space. However, in the gift of the reader's gift, these transformations are of value and potential.

Communicating pain: a process of attunement

Pain is a central element of the hospital experience that exists as a sensation and an emotional experience. But, I find it challenging to describe the role of a painful body sensation or a painful emotional experience in theatre performance because words may not be sufficient to voice the aspects of children's pain. The language of pain is a mystery when emotions are not communicated. Pelander and Leino-Kilpi (2010) argue that most of the worst children's experiences revolve around the concealed, covered and unspoken pain. One of the significant problems with concealed pain is that pain is an unpleasant experience that the child does not always have the language to communicate. The communication of pain in paediatrics is complex because, although language is a powerful communication medium, it is argued that children cannot always find the words to locate and describe their pain. Therefore, pain is not easily shared with adults and healthcare professionals in paediatrics (Carter & Simons 2014). Lascaratou (2007) believes that we should not assume that pain does not exist when pain is not verbalised and that there is no physical and emotional suffering when patients are silent. I think that children may find it challenging to explain their pain. Verbalising pain requires progressive cognitive development and the acquisition of social communication skills that not all children possess. Stanford et al. (2005) argue that self-report in paediatric pain assessment assumes children have acquired a capacity to understand and use common words to describe the pain. How is it assessed and managed if children's pain is not verbalised?

Studies show that children need to develop their language of pain to express verbally how they feel.

> By creating freedom for paediatric patients to experience and convey emotions, the healthcare provider communicates the patient's feelings are valuable and worth listening to and creates an opportunity for deeper connection in the patient-provider relationship. When patients feel understood and validated, they feel safe-mental health professionals call this relational process attunement.
>
> (Julie Lerwick 2016, p. 148)

As in the clinician–patient relationship, attunement is the actor's reactiveness to the child as a participant in theatre activities in the hospital. It is a process of feeling felt, truly listened and cared for by which the actor forms a connection with the child in drama, ideally an empathetic connection. Hepplewhite (2020) discusses empathy in the role of the responsive actor and argues that empathy is a crucial aspect of attunement while attunement is a critical key component of responsivity. Empathy differs from sympathy and an impulse to work with children who suffer from illness. Valuing the social values of practice for participants and themselves, actors enable further connection with individual participants to enrich interactive theatre practice and participants' experience. The actor needs to be aware of the audience's emotional state concerned with feeling, caring imagination and creativity. The ability to experience the same type of emotion as the hospitalised child can be a challenge mainly because the actor's personal experience does not represent the experience of the patient, which can then block the actor's understanding of the child's perspective. Careful interaction between the actor and the child is required so that the child can feel that the actor is tuned in to the child's experience of illness, vulnerability and fragility within a kind and sensitive approach. The actor, for example, can strategically use a gentle approach to connect with the child, which can be a smile or a calm and reassuring body gesture that reveals the actor's nature and personal qualities. The actor must be authentic in what they do. Otherwise, children will immediately sense it and possibly reject the invitation for connection if they feel cheated. But, if the actor is true to themselves, they can encourage children to work synergistically in drama. They can make choices about the end of the story, experiment with objects and their function, and choose a song to sing together. That type of connection appears essential for the actor and the child dynamics, shifting from leader to equal peer with shared ownership of the event. The positioning of the actor needs to be relaxed (take the time for the child to respond), caring (let the child feel listened to and valued) and mindful (be in the present) and encouraging (emphasise the positives) to facilitate empathy, communication and attunement. If empathy is established and communication is achieved, perhaps there will be opportunities for verbalising pain as a form of expression in participatory drama. Thus, improving practices of connection, interaction and communication with hospitalised children through theatre in paediatrics is essential to investigate.

In Erving Goffman's (1959) Dramaturgical Model of social interaction, human social interactions are similar to theatrical roles in performances. Metaphorically speaking, life takes place both on-stage, where actors perform in front of an audience, and backstage, where actors can hide from the audience, resign from their roles and be themselves. In theatrical terms, backstage is the area behind the stage, especially in the dressing rooms. However, Goffman's metaphor, backstage, relates to the theatre people's private lives and inner worlds. Do the stories from hospitalised children illustrate children's personal lives, hidden complicated feelings and pain? Hänninen (2004) suggests a quality to drama in narratives that introduce plots into the flow of knowledge and that narratives represent events and experiences as interconnecting. In this way, meanings can be attributed to experience. Therefore, the reader may want to unpack more about the implicit and explicit fictional stories that children crafted in the face of external difficulties as descriptors of the children's hospital experiences. In doing so, the indirectness of metaphor in some of the stories presented in the book is essential to appreciate. In particular, stories and metaphors are unique in understanding pain (Pugh 1991). Yet, we cannot be precise about what the metaphors in stories reveal regarding how pain is perceived and experienced by children in a clinical setting. Pain is personal and thus relevant. Even when the words exist, children in pain may not find them suitable to portray their feelings. Sepinuck (2013, p. 229) says that 'the *medicine* (in stories) is where the inspiration lies', and the author means the inspiration of the actor and the discovery of joy or comfort in telling their story. Using metaphors may be a way to communicate the physical or emotional pain to others and, by just doing, maybe a way to discover joy. Sometimes finding joy in difficulty is more challenging to do than other times.

Applied theatre or play therapy?

Some of the practices and stories in this book might be described as cathartic, playful and relaxing. The boundaries between artistic and therapeutic approaches can be blurred and bewildering in contexts and settings of illness and vulnerability, such as paediatrics. I distinguish between applied theatre and play therapy with children in hospitals. In my definition, applied theatre in paediatrics is a non-clinical practice that aims to normalise children's hospital experience, entertain and relax them from clinical stressors, improve child wellbeing and maintain their optimism and positivity at times of difficulty through the use of imagination. I previously called applied theatre in paediatrics an 'antidote to clinical stress' that may come with a 'therapeutic potential' (Sextou 2016, p. 32). This is because the ability to enjoy life through the arts during illness can be beneficial and supportive. Play therapy in paediatrics can be applied to the various stages of the medical experience, including both directed and non-directed techniques. Direct play therapy may teach, prepare and support children before, during and after medical procedures. Non-directed therapeutic play occurs when play may be used to identify emotions about their experience of pain (Parson 2008). In therapy, the play's role is to offer children strategies to foster positive growth and effective communication with healthcare staff to maximise clinical benefits. For example, play is used to ease the perioperative anxiety of children, including preparation for anaesthesia (Tonkin 2014). Play therapy comes with a therapeutic intention. Because both applied theatre and play therapy integrate a playful, empathic and curious attitude in cure practices, theatrical interventions may fall into confusion. Further discussion is necessary here to appreciate the value of theatre as an art form and the caring of the actor. He is neither interested nor qualified to treat children's emotional needs and restore their potential traumatic experiences due to illness.

Theatre has been appreciated for its cathartic value for millennia. Aristotle, the Greek polymath, defines tragedy as a means of catharsis and purification. Participating in theatre offers audiences an insight into their lives and opportunities to release negative emotions during the performance. Theatre is meant to provoke feelings connected with recognised problems in the spectator's life by presenting these on the stage, thus allowing the audience to recall and relive them passively and resolve them within the safety of the dramatic representation (Meisiek 2004). Aristotle's definition of tragedy endorses any view that suggests that participating in a play provides the audience with the necessary learning and liberation through the characters' actions. From Boal's point of view (1979), participatory theatre engages audiences actively on stage, offering them the suitable 'space' to think and act on behalf of characters, and the right motivation to reflect on their problems, rehearse their actions and their consequences, and potentially resolve them. Applied theatre can be an excellent educational strategy because it influences the child's personal development, but it cannot promise to cure children (Prentki & Preston 2008); this would be therapy. Brodzinski (2010) argues that applied theatre has a therapeutic approach that gives a chance of a 'healing' experience with particular issues for participants, or it can be the beginning of many reflections. It is the difference between accepting that theatre has the 'therapeutic' *potential* of making the audience feel better and the therapeutic *intention* of using the art form as a tool to cure.

The distinction between *potential* and *intention* is not necessarily a contrasting practice. Applied theatre in paediatrics includes a variety of participatory theatre, storytelling and puppetry practices that are intended to help children enjoy life during illness and improve their wellbeing during treatment. Theatrical interventions are crafted explicitly for audiences who cannot go to the theatre because they are under treatment. In best practice, actors consider the special conditions of space, light, noise, distractions and interruptions in clinical settings and the needs of hospitalised children. Although bedside performance in paediatrics is hosted by healthcare organisations and occurs in clinical settings, the artistic processes and methods do not promise prevention, healing and recovery. They claim no therapeutic benefits even when patients report improved moods, relaxation and engagement with learning (Sextou 2022). Theatre in hospital is primarily an art form focusing on building fictional conditions to achieve characterisation and audience participation in performance. As with all theatre practices, bedside performance in a hospital is often a combination and interlinking of art forms and elements that create that innate sense, feeling or emotion that children cannot easily put into the written and spoken word. It has to do with enjoying being relaxed and playing as a participant in a synergistic performance. Can the arts that children experience during treatment help them cope with stress and deal with their worries better? That is an exciting topic of investigation, but we should not pretend that applied theatre practice, stories and exchanges of emotions have mysterious powers of restoring emotional trauma and curing physical problems. It is essential to recognise that the wellbeing of the hospitalised child is unique to them and intertwined with many other factors in their lives. Especially children with complex medical conditions relocated from their environments and isolated in hospital while undergoing treatment are prone to developing poor social wellbeing. This is timely and important, given the context of the COVID-19 pandemic and its resulting isolation (Sawyer et al. 2021). Their social wellbeing is considerably compromised during their stay in the hospital because it is influenced by the environment around them and the lack of support networks. In paediatrics, where children have become more isolated from friends and family, they may have suffered a shortage of normality, been separated from their siblings, schoolmates and relatives, and, therefore, can lose touch with their social networks. Thus improving hospitalised children's social wellbeing is essential. Being surrounded by actors who treat children with respect in performance can positively affect how children engage and connect with their parents and cooperate with hospital staff to take their medication (Sextou & Hall 2015). However, it is essential to mention that actors are not therapists; thus, differentiating the artistic practice from therapy is necessary.

The significant difference between therapy and applied theatre is the agreement and commitment of the patient to deal with their issues in therapy. The patient in therapy accepts the condition of working persistently, sometimes for periods, to resolve their problems and heal their wounds under the guidance and support of the therapist (Grainger 1995). The problem in this discussion is that little is known about how actors perceive their role in healthcare and its subsequent impact on their relationships with children as audiences both during and after isolation for treatment. It is perilous to perceive their role as healers, therapists, missionaries and good people who sympathise with the ill and suffering and use the arts as a tool to save lives. Frankly, they are actors, servants of the art, trained to make fiction believed as if it is real. In contradiction, my understanding is that therapists are trained to guide the patient, known as the 'client', to use their imagination to transform reality through concentration, deep engagement with the therapeutic process and responsible exploration of their lived experience. Performing under compromised conditions in clinical settings can be emotionally challenging and technically demanding. It is an extraordinary achievement in itself. We must remember that there is a need for appropriate training and ethical research in applied theatre in healthcare, which I will discuss in Chapter 5. To be fair, whatever idea actors may have about their role in the hospital, the understanding of children's struggles is unlikely to be of much success because they are neither trained as psychologists nor therapists. That is expected and entirely understandable. Nevertheless, the tendency to interpret the meaning of applied theatre practice in paediatrics as an intended method for a specific purpose, a 'vehicle' of wellbeing transformation, can mislead a therapeutic attitude and mentality. The actor will engage with the child as a playful participant in the performance, an active audience, rather than as a patient in therapy.

To conclude, applied theatre is not aimed at mending. Just because theatre in a hospital happens in environments of suffering, hope and recovery, it does not mean that bedside performance should be used as a tool for therapy. It can, nevertheless, create empowering conditions for children to improve their wellbeing by communicating what it is like to be as patient. It can also provide hospitalised children with opportunities to look at their realities from a lighter, brighter and less daunting perspective, but only if they come to this learning unintentionally. Therefore, I would encourage the reader to perceive applied theatre in paediatrics and the stories children shared with actors and teachers in this book as important as therapy.

The 'fictional bubble': explosions and interruptions

To better understand the examples in this book, I need to define the role of audiences in paediatrics. Although my bedside participatory theatre model targets hospitalised children in one-to-one interventions, the parents/carers and siblings can get involved as indirect audiences during the performance. I have seen family members reacting to puppets and toys, asking the child questions about the story, interacting with the actor, expressing ideas and making comments. One could observe that indirect audiences intrude in child-centred performances in hospitals designed to focus, prioritise and support the child in a clinical setting. The actor tries to construct a fictional flexible 'bubble', metaphorically speaking, where the child and the actor will be present in a dramatic story. The child steps into the 'bubble' in a non-real, fictional situation, a private condition of a particularly intimate performance. The dramatic conditions of space and time will be protected in the 'bubble' from outside interruptions and disturbances by hospital staff and visitors. The actor always tries to build up trust with the child and secure acceptance of being in the story together by offering a peaceful space for the story to unfold and for the child to relax. In the 'bubble', guided stories can happen through the child's imagination, such as travelling across glittering galaxies in space, playing with a dog on a sandy beach and watching the cherry tree petals dancing in the air-like ballerinas in the spring. Through imagination, the child enters 'the impossible'. Supposing that a flight in space is possible opens a new world of possibilities about things that 'never were, but might become' in drama (Eisen 2006, p. 108). This happens because the success of *telling* the story together results from the child and actor's willing collaboration in the performance process in a private 'fictional bubble' as a metaphor.

In the 'fictional bubble', two situations could become one. For example, a complex reality (I am in bed waiting for surgery) and the imagined situation (there is a lake on a planet far from the Earth) blend into one situation (I am in bed waiting for surgery, but I imagine that I am swimming in a lake in a space cave). In a way, applied theatre in paediatrics becomes the vehicle and the result of blending reality and fiction into one entity, a *metaxis* by-product. The actor's role is to maintain the theatre's aesthetic and remain in the role during the performance, although this can be challenging. Despite the actor's best efforts to connect with the child, the child cannot stay in the fiction for too long, which can be no one's fault. In the absence of a theatrical atmosphere created by the blackout, sound, music and a theatre set, and in the presence of clinical light, images of pain and hospital equipment, it can be very challenging to establish, maintain and reinforce the fictional. The abandonment of the dramatic frame can happen for several reasons. One of them is the indirect audiences. When indirect and uninvited audiences such as parents, caregivers, siblings and healthcare professionals step into the performance, they are reminders of reality and hospitalisation. Interruptions and comments from others, such as 'Oh, that's nice!', 'it's like the toy you play with at home' and 'where did the doggie go?' can explode the fictional 'bubble', break out the dramatic context and completely knock the child out of the fictional frame. Then, the benefits of fictional distraction from ill-related situations are weakened.

Uninvited audiences to intimate performances in hospitals also come with benefits. It is important to remember that bedside performances in paediatrics may become a social event for the whole family. The actor needs to be aware of the widening participation in performance and welcome such engagement as an opportunity for the child to enjoy and normalise their time in the hospital as a family. Sometimes, hospital staff and teachers watch the performance and spontaneously interact with the actor, talk to puppets, respond to artistic objects, express their views and give feedback. Some nurses and teachers are genuinely open to dialogues with the puppets and the children, but their professional focus is different from the actors. However, some comments from parents/caregivers, grandparents and siblings about the intervention are constructive for me to grasp better the role of applied theatre in how families experience child illness in hospitals. Such comments are significant to my learning as authentic feedback. Such witnessing makes the theatrical intervention in the wards more than an artistic activity. It makes it a window for intercultural expression and communication and provides material about the marriage of the two cultures, the artistic and the clinical. Thus, dialogues, reactions and interactions between the actor, the child, the family and hospital staff had not to be ignored in this book.

The act of caring

Caring for applied theatre practice in paediatrics is a way of managing quality care for sick children in clinical services through the arts. There is no specific list of caring tips, but it is essential to recognise that what we care for has nothing to do with how the actors feel when visiting hospitalised children. What lies within the actor is a complex mixture of ideas and responses to illness and the hospital as a space that is charged with specific dominant signs of vulnerability. Caring involves our competence in adjusting to our perception of illness and hospitalisation, if possible. Many actors I worked with carried a strong sense of 'responsibility', of making children happy and relaxed during illness, contained within their experiences with sick children in bedside performances. This may affect their performance profoundly and may require acknowledgement. Mistakenly, actors often carry this overwhelming responsibility unrelated to their role as actors. They, therefore, perceive their role as a hero or heroine in a battle with the difficulty faced by the children. But they cannot help children through the arts if they are living out of mistaken ideas about why children suffer when they are under treatment. Children do not always feel better despite how much the actor offers them in participatory dramas. So for the actor to respond to children as audiences rather than as ill and vulnerable humans, they must challenge the presumptions that limit their understanding of some less obvious factors, other than physical and emotional pain, that affect children's wellbeing when they are in hospital.

Evidence for caring through theatre in children's hospitals shows that the arts can positively impact stress reduction, improving psychological and physiological wellbeing (Sparks 2001; Eisen 2006; Sextou 2016; Lopez-Bushnell & Berg 2018; Astles 2020). These studies demonstrate how art projects in healthcare have provided a valuable means of creating new ways of creative engagement with vulnerable audiences during their stay in the hospital and improving their health. Other studies show that using music (Giordano et al. 2020), illustrated picture books (Yang et al. 2022) and virtual-reality-based simulation (Stunden et al. 2021) can reduce children's pre-operative anxiety and post-operative pain in children undergoing surgery. However, there remains a persistent gap in knowledge and analysis around the deeper meanings and functions of applied theatre in paediatrics as an act of care at times of crisis when family and social support systems fail. With that in mind, further research is needed to examine how emotions are communicated in performance with kindness, compassion, empathy and responsivity during hospitalisation. We need to look at the conditions that need to be in place during a performance for stories to be shared, such as actor professionalism, ethical approach to children and well-framed fictional situations, and how children respond to these conditions. Thus, evaluation of practice is so critical.

The 'marginal participant' technique

Inspired by Hammersley and Atkinson's ethnographic research in practice (2007), I was present in the hospital wards during performances as the leader of projects. The purpose was to watch what happened during the performance about audience participation, listen to what was said and throw light on opportunities for me to learn in a clinical setting. My long experience of applied theatre in medical care settings and my pre-understanding and experience of the context allowed my more in-depth analysis. My presence on the wards aimed to create an opportunity for a deeper analysis of the applied theatre in the paediatrics context and provide me with the potential to better understand the synergies between children and actors. In addition, my focus on audience participation rather than the child's condition aimed to explore the trustworthiness of my bedside performance model, paying attention to possibilities rather than restrictions during illness. There is something quite extraordinary about intimate, spontaneous dialogues involving hospitalised children. This group of children may be vulnerable to the experience of physical pain due to their health conditions. Yet, they can be exceptionally creative, imaginative, responsive and open to synergies. Therefore, I needed to be present during performances to become exposed to various opportunities to learn by witnessing how actors and children interact in practice and develop my competence as a researcher to approach more 'complex' child–actor moments in an intimate performance.

I used the 'marginal participant' technique, in which the researcher plays only a very minimal role in the interaction. I took a non-participating part during performances at Birmingham Children's Hospital and Heartlands Hospital to focus on 'observing' audience participation, what happened in the room or cubicle, how the actor was placed about the child in bed and what interactions and dialogues took place (Ciesielska et al. 2018). While my 'observation' followed a long-time immersion in a specific child healthcare culture as a marginal member conducting non-participant observation, I took the position of an outsider. I tried to distance myself from biased evaluations. Keeping a physical distance to the hospital space used as a 'stage' where the actor and the child meet in the story created opportunities for an objective distancing and witnessing the action. Over the years, I realised that possible reasons for one's acceptance as a non-clinical professional in paediatrics relates to several things, including the family's discomfort with having an outsider there, the child's condition on the day of the performance and the general atmosphere on the ward that can impact on the parents/carers mood and appetite for interaction with unfamiliar others. My decisions about witnessing performances or not were judged on the day and were guided by the parent/carer, the child and the hospital professionals. I made decisions with great sensitivity, ethical awareness and consideration of the difficulties children and families experience in the hospital and their choices and consent to my presence. Either way, it was a great privilege for me to be considered as a marginal participant, a witness and a 'fellow traveller' with them in their journey of illness and recovery.

My learning in a healthcare context was based on the Socratic method of inquiry that is known for its use in philosophy. Still, it is helpful in any discipline with a broad humanistic or liberal arts perspective, as it creates opportunities for self-reflection to encourage critical and imaginative thinking (Mitchell 2006). The Socratic method asks questions rather than providing answers so that learners can discover the complexity and difficulty of specific problems and discover their preconceptions, which may colour their understanding – from a Socratic perspective, witnessing the interactions and interpersonal communications between children, actors and also families of children as indirect audiences allowed me to integrate the experience of others into my learning. The limitation of my reflections on audience participation in a healthcare context is similar to the rules of ethnographic studies in medical students learning in hospitals.

Hägg-Martinell et al. (2017) argue that when the researcher is the tool during observations in clinical settings, research bias and the risk of participants becoming unwilling to act as they would have done if not seen during the performance. Before offering their consent, the children were informed that someone would be standing at a distance to observe the performance, which decreased the risk. If the children or parents/carers preferred not to have an observer in the room or cubicle, I would wait for the actor and the teacher at the ward's reception. On the occasion where consent for me to be present was secured, I would arrive on the ward together with the actor, always escorted by a hospital teacher. While the actor works with the child during the face-to-face performance, I would stand inconspicuously at the back of the room to not distract the child or the actor. I would discreetly reflect on audience participation from a distance without making any contributions, comments or responses. In some cases, I had to stand outside the room and witness through the glass door the children and the actor's movements, body language and non-verbal expressions of feelings such as facial expressions and gestures. On some occasions, children and parents/carers expressed that reflections on the child's entertainment and relaxation were essential and that they wanted to continue with me being present. In other cases, the family did not accept my presence when the child was severely poorly, and I respected that.

In a small way, this book traces the struggle to understand theatre applications and synergies of emotions in paediatrics and areas affected by illness. It aims to explore from my perspective how actors and children as audiences interact in a hospital ward context and how spaces for learning are created and used in such a culture. I will present inspirational examples from the 'Rocket-Arts' and the 'Bird Island' projects and share my notes from before and during the COVID-19 pandemic. My notes are organised by the hospital ward so that the seriousness of the child's condition is recognised in making sense of their struggles and lives. However, my account is part of an attempt to present a taste of the dialogues through synergies of language, ideas, stories and emotions during applied theatre in paediatrics. I aim to offer a way of zooming into intimate and rich, meaningful, improvisatory conversations as a different way of seeing theatre without simplifying the challenges inherent in the practice.

References

Astles, C 2020, 'Walk in/walk as my shoes: Puppetry and prosocial empathy in healthcare', *Journal of Applied Arts and Health*, vol. 11, no. 1–2, pp. 29–47.

Birch, A & Tompkins, J 2012, *Performing Site-Specific Theatre: Politics, Place, Practice*, Palgrave Macmillan: London.

Boal, A 1979, *Theatre of the Oppressed*, Pluto Press: London.

Boal, A 1995, *The Rainbow of Desire: The Boal Method of Theatre and Therapy*, Psychology Press: London.

Boyd, B 2009, *The Origin of Stories. Evolution, Cognition and Fiction*, The Belknap Press Harvard University: Harvard.

Brodzinski, E 2010, *Theatre in Health and Care*, Palgrave Macmillan: London.

Carter, B & Simons, J 2014, *Stories of Children's Pain: Linking Evidence to Practice*, SAGE: London.

Ciesielska, M, Boström, KW & Öhlander, M 2018, 'Observation methods', in M Ciesielska & D Jemielniak (eds), *Qualitative Methodologies in Organization Studies*, Palgrave Macmillan: London.

Eisen, SL 2006, *The Healing Effects of Art in Pediatric Healthcare: Art Preferences of Healthy Children and Hospitalised Children*, PhD thesis, Texas A&M University: College Station, TX.

Gallagher, MW, Lopez, SJ & Preacher, KJ 2009, 'The hierarchical structure of well-being', *Journal of Personality*, vol. 77. https://doi.org/10.1111/j.1467-6494.2009.00573.x.

Giordano, F, Zanchi, B, De Leonardis, F, Rutigliano, C, Esposito, F, Brienza, N & Santoro, N 2020, 'The influence of music therapy on preoperative anxiety in pediatric oncology patients undergoing invasive procedures', *The Arts in Psychotherapy*, vol. 68. https://doi.org/10.1016/j.aip.2020.101649.

Goffman, E 1959, The presentation of self in everyday life. *Doubleday*. https://monoskop.org/images/1/19/Goffman_Erving_The_Presentation_of_Self_in_Everyday_Life.pdf

Gottschall, J 2012, *The Storytelling Animal: How Stories Make us Human*, Mifflin Harcourt: Houghton.

Grainger, R 1995, *Drama and Healing. The Roots of Dramatherapy*, Jessica Kingsley Publishers: London.

Hägg-Martinell, A, Hult, H & Henriksson, P 2017, 'Medical students opportunities to participate and learn from activities at an internal medicine ward: An ethnographic study', *BMJ Open*, vol. 7. https://bmjopen.bmj.com/content/7/2/e013046.

Hammersley, M & Atkinson, P 2007, *Ethnography: Principles in Practice*, Routledge: London.

Hänninen, V 2004, 'A model of narrative circulation', *Narrative Inquiry*, vol. 14, no. 1. www.jbe-platform.com/content/journals/10.1075/ni.14.1.04han.

Hepplewhite, K 2020, *The Applied Theatre Actor. Responsivity and Expertise in Practice*, Palgrave Macmillan: London.

Howell, C, Cox, S, Drew, S, Guillemin, M, Warr, D & Waycott, J 2015, 'Exploring ethical frontiers of visual methods', *Research Ethics*, vol. 10, no. 4. https://doi/10.1177/1747016114552685.

Jackson, A 2007, *Theatre, Education and the Making of Meanings, Art or Instrument?*, Manchester University Press: Manchester.

Lascaratou, C 2007, *The Language of Pain*, Jon Benjamins Publishing Company: Philadelphia, PA.

Lerwick, JL 2016, 'Minimizing pediatric healthcare-included anxiety and trauma', *World Journal of Clinical Pediatrics*, vol. 5, no. 2. https://pubmed.ncbi.nlm.nih.gov/27170924/.

Lindon, J 2002, *What is Play?*, Children's Play Information Service National Children's Bureau: London.

Lopez-Bushnell, F & Berg, M 2018, 'Effects of art experience on hospitalised pediatric patients', *Matthews Journal of Pediatrics*, vol. 3, no. 1. www.mathewsopenaccess.com/full-text/effects-of-art-experience-on-hospitalised-pediatric-patients.

Meisiek, S 2004, 'Which Catharsis do they mean? Aristotle, Moreno, Boal and organisation theatre', *Organisation Studies*, vol. 25, no. 5. https://doi.org/10.1177/0170840604042415.

Mitchell, S 2006, 'Socratic dialogue, the humanities and the art of the question', *Arts and Humanities in Higher Education*, vol. 5, no. 2. https://eric.ed.gov/?id=EJ793133.

O'Toole, J 1992, *The Process of Drama: Negotiating Art and Meaning*, Routledge: London.

Parson, J 2008, *Integration of Procedural Play for Children undergoing Cystic Fibrosis Treatment: A Nursing Perspective*, Central Queensland University: Queensland.

Pascal, B 1669, *Pensées*. www.artandpopularculture.com/Pens%C3%A9es.

Pelander, T & Leino-Kilpi, H 2010, 'Children's best and worst experiences during hospitalisation', *Scandinavian Journal of Caring Sciences*, vol. 24, no. 4. https://doi.org/10.1111/j.1471-6712.2010.00770.x.

Prentki, T & Preston, S 2008, *The Applied Theatre Reader*, Routledge: London.

Pugh, JF 1991, 'The semantics of pain in Indian culture and medicine', *Culture, Medicine and Psychiatry*, vol. 15, no. 1. https://doi.org/10.1007/bf00050826.

Saint-Exupéry, A. 1943, *The Little Prince*, (First Edition), Reynal & Hitchcock: New York.

Sakr, Y, Moreira, CL, Rhodes, A, Ferguson, ND, Kleinpell, R, Pickkers, P, Kuiper, MA, Lipman, J & Vincent, JL 2015, 'Extended prevalence of infection in intensive care study investigators. The impact of hospital and ICU organizational factors on outcome in critically ill patients: results from the extended prevalence of infection in intensive care study', *Critical Care Medicine*, vol. 43, no. 3. doi: 10.1097/CCM.0000000000000754. PMID: 25479111.

Sawyer, JL, Mishna, F, Bouffet, E & Work, J 2021, 'Bridging the gap: Exploring the impact of hospital isolation on peer relationships among children and adolescents with a malignant brain tumor', *Child and Adolescent Social Work Journal*. https://doi.org/10.1007/s10560-021-00764-x.

Sepinuck, T 2013, *Theatre of Witness: Finding the Medicine in Stories of Suffering, Transformation, and Peace*, Jessica Kingsley Publisher: London.

Sextou, P 2016, *Theatre for Children in Hospital. The Gift of Compassion*, Intellect: Bristol.

Sextou, P 2022, 'Theatre in paediatrics: Can participatory performance mitigate educational, emotional and social consequences of missing out school during hospitalisation?', *Research in Drama Education: The Journal of Applied Theatre and Performance*, vol. 27, no. 1. https://doi.org/10.1080/13569783.2021.1940914.

Sextou, P & Hall, S 2015, 'Hospital theatre promoting child wellbeing in cardiac and cancer units', *Applied Theatre Research*, vol. 3, no. 1, pp. 67–84.

Sextou, P & Hall, S 2015, 'Theatre & community: Bedside theatre promoting child wellbeing in cardiac and cancer units', *Applied Theatre Research*, vol. 3, no. 1. www.academia.edu/8667175/

Sparks, L 2001, 'Taking the "ouch" out of injections for children: Using distraction to decrease pain', *American Journal of Maternal/Child Nursing*, vol. 26, pp. 72–78.

Stanford, EA, Chambers, CT & Craig, KD 2005, 'A normative analysis of the development of pain-related vocabulary in children', *Pain*, vol. 114, no. 1–2. https://doi.org/10.1016/j.pain.2004.12.029.

Stunden, C, Stratton K, Zakani, S & Jacob J 2021, 'Comparing a Virtual Reality-Based Simulation App (VR-MRI) with a standard preparatory manual and child life program for improving success and reducing anxiety during pediatric medical imaging: randomized clinical trial', *Journal of Medical Internet Research*, vol. 23, no. 9. www.jmir.org/2021/9/e22942.

Thompson, J 2005, *Digging up Stories. Applied Theatre, Performance and War*, Manchester University Press: Manchester.

Thompson, J 2012, *Applied Theatre: Bewilderment and Beyond*, Peter Lang: Oxford.

Tonkin, A 2014, The provision of play in health service delivery fulfilling children's rights under Article 31 of the United Nations Convention on the Rights of the Child. A literature review. *National Association of Health Play Specialists*. www.england.nhs.uk/6cs/wp-content/uploads/sites/25/2015/03/nahps-full-report.pdf.

Yang, Y, Zhang, M, Sun, Y, Peng, Z, Zheng, X & Zheng, J 2022, 'Effects of advance exposure to an animated surgery-related picture book on preoperative anxiety and anaesthesia induction in preschool children: A randomised control trial', *BMC Paediatrics*, vol. 22, no. 92. https://doi.org/10.1186/s12887-022-03136-1.

2
APPLIED THEATRE AND DIGITAL ASSETS ON THE WARDS

In this chapter, I am sharing 'Rocket-Arts', a specific example of my bedside theatre practice in the hospital that uses a combination of media, including storytelling performances, experimental work with puppets and objects such as miniature Playmobil toys, a portable space rocket 3D installation, and digital toy-based films as resources. I will briefly present the project to illustrate the challenges and rewards of navigating the 'Rocket-Arts' through the turbulences of the COVID-19 pandemic when healthcare systems collapsed. I introduce the pre-pandemic bedside performance and the post-pandemic digital solutions phases of the 'Rocket-Arts' project to argue that applied theatre in paediatrics can resist the restriction of only one approach, model and method. It must be open to new vocabularies, media and deliveries. This chapter is aimed to set up the conditions and prepare the audience for reading the stories I am presenting in Chapter 3. Therefore, I will offer information for the reader to position the method of collecting stories and the stories children told in response to the 'Rocket-Arts' project within the context of illness, artistry, creativity and learning. Descriptions of the setting, the story's content, the materials and the media we used aim to transport the reader to hospital wards. This will have a significance for thinking of the need for constant improvisation and improvement of practice in experimentation with art forms, techniques and materials, a process of enlightening and professional development.

The 'Rocket-Arts' project in hospitals

'Rocket-Arts' was implemented in multiple wards of children's hospitals within the National Health System (NHS) in England between 2019 and 2021. The project aimed to make a difference in child patients' social and emotional wellbeing and improve their engagement with creative activities and education during their treatment. 'Rocket-Arts' tells the story of Simba, the therapy dog, and a little boy in the hospital. Simba, our family red cocker spaniel, inspired me to write a storybook for children in the hospital undergoing treatment and for children who are poorly at home or feel lonely and need a friend to escape to places by using their imagination. In the script (Appendix A), I place the story's beginnings in a clinical environment when a boy is admitted to a hospital. A boy is taken to the scan room to undergo magnetic resonance imaging (MRI) of the brain used for diagnostic purposes. During his admission to the hospital, the boy meets with Simba, a therapy dog, and they connect immediately. Once the boy and Simba become friends, they get on a space rocket and head to explore space. Their travelling from planet to planet happens in a 'dream' mode when the boy in the story is under sedation to undergo an MRI. In their dream, the boy and the dog fly into galaxies like pink and purple rivers, where they meet space animals, a wolf, a fox, a cat and a phoenix, a beautiful bird symbolising rebirth and eternal life. Space animals become glittering star constellations in the black universe. Everything in space is very peaceful, but the boy and the dog want to return to Earth. A spacecraft picks them up just on time and lands them back in the hospital in the exact spot where the story started in the scan room. The scan procedure is over when the two characters return to the hospital. To everyone's surprise, a phoenix flies across the room, scattering space dust particles in the shape of confetti.

We told the children about Simba's adventures in space, aiming to distract children, relax their minds and mitigate their experience of anxiety in anticipation of a clinical procedure (Appendix A: the script). I wrote Simba's story to explore the effectiveness of theatrical, non-pharmaceutical interventions in counteracting stress and assess whether such interventions might relax the child before an MRI. Many children undergo a scan, and although the process is not painful, it requires them to remain still for approximately 45 min. Viggiano et al. (2015) argue that children undergoing MRI examinations frequently experience negative emotions such as anxiety and fear before and during the scanning. Consequently, the children cannot remain still during the procedure. Since obtaining a motion-free MRI scan can be challenging for children, sedation is sometimes necessary. Although the story does not directly address pain, physical or emotional, pain is acknowledged as an experience. The characters, such as a boy patient, his father, the doctor, the dog's trainer and Simba, all know the pain experienced as a sensation and an emotion. 'Rocket-Arts' audience numbers reached approximately 3,600 vulnerable children, aged 5–11, affected by illness or injury and their siblings. It is important to remember that children in healthcare are audiences to actors rather than patients. The project was offered to long-term hospital children suffering from chronic health conditions and behavioural and emotional difficulties. These children may feel less confident about communicating and managing emotions effectively and will need additional support to adapt to routine changes and understand what is going on in their lives when support systems collapse (The Children's Society 2021). 'Rocket-Arts' was implemented in two phases, pre- and post-COVID-19, opening me to new possibilities because of the pandemic.

Pre-pandemic bedside performance

Phase one involved face-to-face bedside performances on hospital wards across the Women and Children's Birmingham NHS Trust and the Heart of England Foundation NHS Trust between October 2019 and March 2020. We met children in different wards, including participants in nephrology, dialysis, oncology, paediatric surgery, cardiac, neurosurgery, the burns centre and general paediatrics. I worked closely with professional actors and installation artists. They explored using art recycled materials, drama, improvisation, puppetry, object animation and storytelling during rehearsals to engage children. One-to-one participatory activities were implemented bedside. An actress landed a 6.5-foot high and 1.6-foot diameter portable space rocket attached to a four-hook intravenous drip stand base on the hospital ward.

Following NHS hygiene regulations, the base of the space rocket was manufactured from stainless steel to be hygienic and easy to clean. The stand hooks were easy to adjust, providing optimum transportation throughout the hospital environment. The top of the space rocket was made of a recycled barrel with doors that kept the interior as a surprise to the child until the doors opened to reveal two compartments. Each compartment created a miniature 'stage' allowing space to position a selection of Playmobil toy figures. Children animated miniature toys (Playmobil astronauts, robots, explorers, spaceships, etc.) and got involved in story-making activities by using spontaneous oral speech as they do in their play.

The rocket prop was inspired by the concept of a miniature Victorian Toy Theatre, popular children's toys until their decline at the end of the nineteenth century. Miniature stages, characters, scenery and props were printed onto paper from copper plates and sold by publishers and stationers as individual sheets. These could be cut out, pasted onto cards and painted. The 'actors' were mounted onto little tin slides and were pushed onto the stage from the side wings (Honey 2018). For the many Victorian toys, theatres may only offer us nostalgia for past times today. However, I think it also provides us with a model of a portable stage that reveals a dream world to participant audiences. The model of miniature theatre for the needs of 'Rocket-Arts' was a solution for creating a 'stage' in confined spaces such as the limited space where bedside performances happen on hospital wards.

I observed in my practice that when a child is in a hospital bed, their personal space, the child's body and possessions come to a public display—they are genuinely shared. This sharing is complex and often uncomfortable. Privacy, and sometimes dignity, is seriously negotiated. Illness reconstructs the child's experience of personal and private life in particular ways on a hospital ward; there is the strangeness of realising that unfamiliar adults get to see the child in their pyjamas or without them, and, in this regard, the ownership of the space around the bed is shown to be compromised. Therefore, the artist is asked and should be trained to visit the child's bedside with respect, caution and discretion. The artist needs to enable the child to have the confidence to decide the proximity, to show them where to stand concerning their private space for the boundaries between the personal and the public to be identified and respected.

In Chapter 1, I discussed the investment in creating opportunities for the child to connect with the actor in a fictional 'bubble' and the importance of the space in-between fiction and reality, clinical and metaphorical. In 'Rocket-Arts', once the space between the child in bed and the actor on the chair bedside is symbolised as 'stage', the two of them imagine themselves entering the fictional dimensions of aerospace. The physical space becomes a department where a spacecraft is constructed. The portable spacecraft is placed next to the child's bed, inviting the child to converse with the environment. Because of the emotional significance of the space bedside in the hospital, entering that space as an actor is a delicate experience – the invasion of personal freedom and the process of being accepted in that confined space by a child is essential to the performance. The status of the space as 'property' of the bed owner, the symbol of the identity of the ill person and the power of that space in addressing the child's isolation and seclusion from the rest of the world is remarkable. It is tough to ignore the vibes of illness in the space and the dominant messages of pain and suffering in a clinical setting. However, it is virtually impossible that a portable space rocket of 6.5-foot height cannot attract the child's attention and distract its mind from the surroundings. My experience of witnessing children while watching the entrance of the space rocket on the ward and then opening its doors to a world of miniature toys is part of this argument. We introduced children to Playmobil toys such as astronauts, explorers, princesses and princes, rock singers, dogs and unicorns, all positioned within the space rocket, waiting for the children to animate them as tiny actors on elaborated sets. However, the object theatre started creating its meaning once the actor opened a box with a different setup. In the box, the hospital setting and patients as characters were replicated by Playmobil toys.

Toy theatre was taken to the bedside, hoping it would also become alive in the little fingers of hospitalised children as if they were real characters on a theatre stage. For many children, Playmobil toys are those familiar objects that are personal belongings. Therefore, it was aimed that toys will become very much alive during the story, offering children opportunities to escape to imagined worlds – ones not available anywhere else – during their hospitalisation. Children animated the small bodies as if they were playing with them in their own home. It felt that familiarity with toys in 'Rocket-Arts' added a sense of normality to the hospital experience. It felt as if the rocket and the toys provided children with a focus by attracting their attention to its interior, enabling them to 'zoom in' to a Lilliputian scenery where proportions differ from reality. Thus, the escape into the fictional world can happen. It is similar to the effect of the darkroom when we visit cinemas. All that matters in the darkness is the source of light, the moving image that brings things other than what we know to live in front of our own eyes and, for a moment or two, create the illusion that what is not natural can be believed as if it is accurate.

The performer was flexible and open to changes as a mindful practice required in healthcare settings (Ashford 2019). Although there is a script for the actor, my bedside model is located within a practice of free improvisation where the actor becomes a narrator who presents a narrative thread to the child that can be adapted to the child's suggestions. Simba's story was performed 'within the freedom to oscillate between a controlled performance using a script and an improvised performance led by a storyline'. Fitzpatrick (1995, p. 48) defines flexible performance 'as a mode of performance in which the performer has the liberty to generate with some flexibility actions and words appropriate to the context and their sources to do so in a coherent, pertinent, and acceptable way'. This model encourages an inter-play between the elements of the role and personal resources and allows the actor to generate a synergistic performance in response to their audience for the child to contribute and lead action. The performance was open to possible starters and different endings based on the agreement between the actor and the child. The general storyline was followed throughout, subject to the child's appetite and the ability for inter-play.

Performances were accommodated on the hospital wards with assistance from a committed team of ten hospital teachers. I involved hospital teachers in using the teacher's intuitive skills and educational abilities (Csinády 2015) to engage with children in non-clinical activities. Hospital teachers were chosen to accommodate the project on the wards because of their unique position about children's experience of play and learning, both naturally related to normality, and their knowledge and understanding of facilitating creative activities effectively in a hospital setting. Guidance was included in the research protocol and was approved by my institution. Guidance for the teachers involved instructions about safeguarding and respecting the child as a participant. Teachers were also offered advice about the provision of withdrawal options and clear directions to avoid the habit of correcting children's language during participation in performance and keep the freshness and originality of children's stories. Hospital teachers were selected by the Head of school and had no personal relationship with me, although collaborations between myself and the school had taken place previously. This experience of knowing teachers' professionalism, responsibility and moral commitment to working with children in line with the hospital's safeguarding policies during COVID-19 reassured me.

Post-pandemic digital solutions

Phase two was developed from phase one between March 2020 and March 2021. Following news developments relating to the COVID-19 pandemic and having closely followed advice and guidance from the government, the World Health Organisation and Public Health England, and NHS, the 'Rocket-Arts' project had to pause performances on the hospital wards from March 2020 until June 2020. Actors were not allowed to visit hospitals (unfortunately, this is still the case in England). Therefore, creative ways had to be implemented to enable sick children to access the arts remotely during unprecedented times. Films targeted children in three age groups (5–6, 7–8 and 9–11 years) and lasted approximately 5 min each. We used theatre and performance principles and digital media examples as tools for telling Simba's stories with the little boy in space. We shared ideas and potential cartoon images with family friends with children in the targeted age groups. Their preferences were encountered in the materials we gathered. We explored a variety of potential assets, such as pictures of Simba, digital backgrounds or music, before choosing an aesthetic for each film.

The films of phase two grew out of the storytelling of phase one, but each film's animation type varied. We worked in many kinds of animation, including 2D and 3D animation, motion graphics, collage and stop motion techniques. For example, in the film 'Here I am flying!' (Sextou 2020), we took photographs of each new position to move Playmobil toys as objects physically (Appendix B: adaptation of performance in a digital film). We created an illusion of movement when the pictures were played in sequence. To imagine Simba in space with astronauts and robots in motion, we set up tableaux, frozen scenes with the same space rocket that toured the wards and the same set of miniature toys (Playmobil) and puppets children animated. We took pictures of the tableaux scene-by-scene and used them in the film to create a storyline. This choice aimed to establish a connection between the project's two phases and produce movies based on toys that children are familiar with. In phase one, children took physical possession of the toys as part of their private property for personal use in drama. In phase two, children watched the cartoon and toy-based films. All children were offered new Playmobil sets to keep in their possession in both phases. They could animate their toy while watching the movie (s), play with it afterwards, use it to recall the film experience with the teacher while making a story or keep it as a memoir. 'Rocket-Arts' E-resources played through the James Brindley Academy's website for the children in-patients at Birmingham Children's Hospital and their ex-patient pupils experiencing isolation at home. They were also accessible to the broader public via my institution's website. With a small team of hospital teachers working remotely, we produced a selection of online worksheet literacy activities resources for children during successive lockdowns.

Films were played, and stories were collected with assistance from a committed team of hospital teachers based on the belief that children's behaviour and attitude can better be discovered and explored through gathering facts from experience, observation and experimentation (Wisker 2009). Hospital teachers downloaded the films on their devices. Children chose to watch as many of those films as they wanted (all or none) depending on their mood, abilities and needs. Children watched the downloaded files on the school's approved devices together at their teacher's bedside. Following the film, teachers offered children a set of story-making activities (15–20 min) where they could use their imagination to tell their own stories for a little out-of-this-world escape to keep them occupied and creative during their stay in hospital.

Collection of stories

Hospital teachers followed up the 'Rocket-Arts' bedside intervention on the same day after the actor left the ward during phase one to create opportunities for the child to use the raw experience of performance as a stimulus for making a story of their own.

Before implementing the project, I facilitated a workshop for the hospital school teaching staff to guide their follow-up role and answer their questions.

The teachers were invited to think about how the arts, when shared ethically and respectfully with the hospitalised child, might enable the expression of personal experience and emotions verbally. I also cared to explain that the performance intended to create a space where all experiences of vulnerability, impairment and disability are valid. Stories were documented on a proforma that I specially designed for the project. The proforma offered space for children to write a story using a flexible story-making guide (Howitt & Cramer 2017) and draw a picture about their favourite character or themselves in the story. To elicit unstructured responses and generate an appetite for writing a story inspired by 'Rocket-Arts', a mixture of 'probe' sentence starters was used on the proforma (McIntosh & Morse 2015). Children could select one of the following indicative opening sentences.

> Once upon a time, there was a monster sitting outside a spaceship . . .
> The astronaut looked out of the window of this spaceship to see the moon had changed colour . . .
> The two friends entered a space cave when they heard a loud crashing noise . . .
> 'What a beautiful garden,' the Princess whispered . . .
> A unicorn showed up just at the right time . . .

Indicative starters were followed by a dedicated space of ten lines where the child could write their own story. When necessary, hospital teachers assisted the children with writing. The teacher's guidance was to use the child's words and avoid paraphrasing. After the performance, some questions naturally emerged from the dialogue between children and hospital teachers (Berg 1989). These illustrate how the experience of participating in the arts engaged the audience by telling stories and communicating feelings.

> Where do you think that . . . happened?
> How many animals/diamonds etc., are hidden in the . . .?
> What happened to . . . after they . . .?
> Where do you want . . . to go?
> How do . . . feel about the . . .?
> Can you see yourself in the story? Where?

Making a story aimed to be open, flexible and engaging because for children in the hospital to communicate their feelings, they need the confidence to use the stimuli we offer them in performance. It can be tough to describe one's experience without supporting materials such as the use of the context and vocabulary of performance. Following the input of the adult, children were free to get inspiration from the performance, deconstruct the story, use elements of it or not, add new ideas, characters and feelings, reconstruct the story in different possible scenarios and try to express their subjective experience of being in hospital in their own words.

Young children (aged 3–6) told their stories to the teachers, who wrote them down on their proforma. Older children (aged 7–11), who were more confident with writing, wrote their stories directly on the proforma. Some children presented developmental delays subject to long-term hospitalisation. Children with recurrent admissions can be at greater risk for experiencing regression to lower developmental stages (Cahayag 2020). With the possible effects of long-term hospitalisation on children's development, the performance encouraged children to use their senses in the story by offering them sensory scaffolds such as visuals, gestures, music and puppets. How each child responded to those stimuli, assimilated, accommodated and adapted the story may differ. For example, some of the stories grew naturally out of the performance. Children based their narratives on the memory of what they saw and how they used toys to interact with the actor and duplicated parts, if not all, of the story plot as it evolved during the performance. Some children recalled whole dialogues from the story. Some stories 'recycled' words and expressions from the actor's vocabulary during the performance. Other children produced novel and stimulating material. Characters, places and feelings were described, such as 'the princess and the prince was lifted to the sky', 'an astronaut was scared' and 'wellies were happy'. Other stories moved away from the performance 'memories', showing some ownership levels of the activity.

On one occasion, for example, the child told us this story.

A star was lonely in space. The star travelled days and nights to get closer to the Earth. The star could see a safari group lost in the jungle. The star got closer to light up the sky for the safari group to find their way back.

Without bedside performance, we would have less access to this child's vibrant imagination. However, the translation of what the child meant by this story is complex because each child has a different 'emotional lexicon' that describes incidents and communicates feelings. Emotion vocabulary development poses specific challenges as the domain of emotions is defined less clearly than those of tangible objects or perceivable features (Grosse et al. 2021). Therefore, it is unclear how the child used their emotional lexicon to describe feelings of loneliness. However, we cannot rule out the possibility that the child provided us with a description of the emotional needs they experienced because they could supplement their verbal description with recollections from the performance. As applied theatre practitioners and healthcare professionals working with children, we need to take stories seriously because these stories are what we have available to use and to understand, or assume that we know better how children feel. Translation and interpretation of stories deserve attention and thoughtfulness. The levels represent the sick child's journey from being a passive patient and recipient of the arts to becoming an active participant and co-creator of the arts in the hospital. In other words, it symbolises the effective transformation of identity from the 'ill and unable to do' to the 'ill and able to do' child who can tell stories and enjoy life during times of discomfort.

The impact of COVID-19 on 'Rocket-Arts'

With 'Rocket-Arts' as an example, applied theatre in paediatrics can resist a single approach, model and method, and be open to new vocabularies, media and deliveries. This gives me a challenge as a researcher. COVID-19 came to my world to promote a whole other world of possibilities for my practice. I was new to digital technology and experiencing challenges settling into the idea of not being allowed to lead face-to-face applied theatre performances in hospitals. But, by drawing on other people's knowledge and experience in digital films, I navigated myself through the turbulences of sailing in unknown waters. I facilitated the possibility of developing alternative tools for reaching out to children in need by altering the focus between each expertise. The key to adapting to the circumstances is being open to new forms and media and critical of the process unfolding. 'Rocket-Arts' aimed to bring children into a fantasy world where they could celebrate moments of engagement with the arts. Inviting children to participate in fictional stories encouraged them to experience new places within their hospital lives and create fewer illness-related experiences. The child and the actor could have shared ownership. This example shows how openness to experimentation with forms and techniques enables a researcher to move from *relying on expertise* to *experimenting with expertise*. By interacting with actors and digital actors, I was made aware of the boundaries in life between safety within the tested and known and new attempts where the learning requires a leap of faith in the unknown. It is a moment of understanding the language of modesty. It was an act of certainty due to the pandemic, of course.

During this transition, the focus on the child as a spectator in response to ethics, care and responsibility remained. The participatory performance and the digital films, although in different forms, reflect a precise alignment to the care context through the aesthetics, caring choices of approaches, materials and words. Thompson (2015, p. 437) defines the aesthetics of care as 'a form of crafted caring where learning to create, respond and be in close dialogue with others is vital for the quality of the experience: but it is a "temporally extensive form" because it needs to be "continuously modified" as it is practised'. My experimentation with art forms, techniques and materials coincides with Thompson's suggestion for constant improvisation and improvement of practice. 'Rocket-Arts' offered me opportunities for improvisation, identification of weaknesses and problems in practice, and investigation of alternative methods of delivery and presentation process and enlightening. It was effective because it improved my learning and helped me grow familiarity with self-observation. What for me was confident practice for many years had to be rediscovered as an emergency due to the pandemic. In this journey of discovery, one can accept imperfection as less critical to new learnings and raise questions about the boundaries between disciplines. How do we develop an awareness of multi-disciplinary practice to fit for purpose? How do we create an understanding of our practice, and how do we reinvent, recreate and rework our attitudes towards our flaws and failings?

Perhaps the most critical learning from 'Rocket-Arts' was to find the strength to fight for my value as a human being and pursue eudaimonia actions. This asks to question of whether good actions are actions of selfishness or altruism. This asks where passion for applied theatre in paediatrics begins and where it stops. This asks how can expertise and experience be combined across disciplines for the benefit of the community and where arts-based principles and technological development are achieved. The next step should be to examine the cross-disciplinary tensions and aim for more elaborated synergies of compassion, looking for similarities and differences and ways of co-existence and responsiveness.

References

Ashford, L 2019, 'The flexible performer in applied theatre: In-hospital interaction with captain Starlight', *ArtsPraxis*, vol. 6, no. 2. www.researchgate.net/publication/343901471_The_Flexible_Performer_in_Applied_Theatre_In-_hospital_Interaction_with_Captain_Starlight_ArtsPraxis_62.

Berg, BL 1989, *Qualitative Research Methods for the Social Science*, Allyn and Bacon: Toronto.

Cahayag, V 2020, 'Hospitalization and child development: Effects on sleep, developmental stages, and separation anxiety', *Nursing | Senior Theses*, vol. 17. https://doi.org/10.33015/dominican.edu/2020.NURS.ST.09.

Csinády, R 2015, 'Hospital pedagogy, a bridge between hospital and school', *Hungarian Educational Research Journal*, vol. 5, no. 2, pp. 49–65.

Fitzpatrick, T 1995, *The Relationship of Oral and Literate Performance Processes in the Commedia Dell'arte: Beyond the Improvisation/Memorisation Divide*, Edwin Mellen Press: Lewiston.

Grosse, G, Streubel, B, Gunzenhauser, C & Saalbach, H 2021, 'Let's talk about emotions: The development of children's emotion vocabulary from 4 to 11 years of age', *Affective Science*, vol. 2. https://doi.org/10.1007/s42761-021-00040-2.

Honey, L 2018, *The History of Antique Toy Theatres*, Homes & Antiques Publication. https://www.homesandantiques.com/antiques/collecting-guides-antiques/experts/antique-toy-theatres-make-the-best-scenes/.

Howitt, D & Cramer, D 2017, *Research Methods in Psychology*, Pearson: London.

McIntosh, MJ & Morse, JM 2015, 'Situating and constructing diversity in semi-structured interviews', *Global Qualitative Nurse Research*, vol. 14, no. 2. https://doi.org/10.1177/2333393615597674.

Sextou, P 2020, *'Here I am flying!' bespoke animated film for children in hospital*. www.youtube.com/watch?v=azF6HlI0r2w&t=27s.

The Children's Society 2021, *The impact of COVID-19 on children and young people*. www.childrenssociety.org.uk/sites/default/files/2021-01/the-impact-of-COVID-19-on-children-and-young-people-briefing.pdf.

Thompson, J 2015, 'Towards an aesthetics of care', *Research in Drama Education: The Journal of Applied Theatre and Performance*, vol. 20, no. 4. https://doi.org/10.1080/13569783.2015.1068109.

Viggiano, MP, Giganti, F, Rossi, A, Di Feo, D, Vagnoli, L, Calcagno, G & Defilippi, C 2015, 'Impact of psychological interventions on reducing anxiety, fear and the need for sedation in children undergoing magnetic resonance imaging', *Pediatric Reports*, vol. 7, no. 1. www.ncbi.nlm.nih.gov/pmc/articles/PMC4387329/.

Wisker, G 2009, *The Undergraduate Research Handbook*, Palgrave Macmillan: London.

3
SICK CHILDREN'S STORIES
From patients to story-makers

This chapter presents genuine, humorous and joyful stories of hospitalised children in response to applied theatre practice. As I have witnessed these stories myself, I have tried to reflect on the incidents trying to honour the children who participated in the project. Each story is followed by my observations on the synergies between the child and the artists and personal reflections. Still, my reflections are a tiny fragment of what I witnessed on hospital wards and how I understand how each child experienced the applied theatre. The selection of stories was beyond the scope of evaluating the children's creations – but decisions were made to create a sense of worth in children's struggles. It will be up to the reader to see the significance of that display. The chapter also offers a critical discussion about the symbolic space where the stories evolved, a 'stitched land' between fiction and hospital reality. It concludes that participatory performance creates opportunities for children to move from the identity of being an ill and unable patient to being a sick and able child by a shift of power that restores agency to children. Applied theatre in paediatrics offers experiences with an appropriate balance of challenges relating to understanding emotions and protection provided by the context of fiction. Because stories in paediatrics are powerful in affecting both minds and hearts, when you read these stories, allow some time to engage with them and prepare to be involved.

Introduction to stories

At the heart of applied theatre in paediatrics is storytelling. Although humans are sophisticated beings, we have difficulty expressing and communicating feelings. But children are compulsive creators of pretended events that recombine elements of reality and fantasy stepping over the actual into the possible, the imagined and, sometimes, the impossible. Thus, children can tell stories without acting them out

DOI: 10.4324/9781003039341-3

(Boyd 2009). Adults could learn to communicate emotions with children more efficiently by paying attention to how children tell stories. To further understand how children feel and what they say when participating in one-to-one performances during their stay in the hospital, the actor needs to shift their focus from the outcome (the story as a final product) to the process and engage with the child and the environment. The engagement with children in performance and varied and complex conceptualisations in stories also create a need to attend to how children and actors exchange emotions. Because stories are active and resourceful and theatre provides participants with metaphor, actors and children in paediatrics 'walk' into the fiction together where feelings are shared either directly or indirectly. Nevertheless, the journey of knowing about children and interacting with them in times of illness can be elusive.

Stories of this book are creations of verbal improvisation with puppets, playmobile toys and objects in confined spaces in healthcare contexts. They are products of the actor–child relationship, active listening, improvisation, patience, attention to senses and willingness to compassionate communication and empathic understanding. Each story expresses unique moments of children's imagination, all valuable in revealing how important it is to attend to artistic expression. Theatre is nothing if not an art form enacted within possibility. I place children, stories and the phenomenon of emotions within applied theatre in healthcare to pose critical questions about the role of performing stories in hospitals and the best approach to creating possibilities for audience participation in exploratory worlds. I am observant as being present in practice as part of the research. I write as a reflective practitioner who draws upon theory to make meaning of practice and understand the emotions in practice. Taken from my lengthy research and practice experience in hospitals and hospices, I explore the link between performance, entertainment, education and wellbeing in child healthcare. I see stories through an unconventional lens about how children and actors engage in conversations in performance, taking note of the dialogue and the body language, the silences, and the actor and nurse's interruptions. I use all the senses offering intimate details to describe the levels of participation in the story, transporting the reader to the moment and into the story. My value systems, professional and life experiences have been kept separate from proofreading so that each story's writing style and truth are represented without any meaningful alterations. The stories are presented to inspire, motivate and facilitate discussion and further understanding of participatory drama approaches and artistic processes in healthcare. I ask if the stories continue as extensions of the children, providing means to understand aspects of the children's language of emotions in hospital life. I am interested in how bespoke one-to-one performances are perceived, conceived, recreated and reinvented by the child, the actor and the professional hospital teachers. This will raise questions about whether bedside performance in hospitals inspires participants and offers them a pre-text to build on their stories.

The collection of stories took place at a Children's Hospital in England within a research study following institutional ethical approvals, and it complied with the hospital and school safeguarding policies and codes of ethical practice. The selected stories have been edited by myself, focusing on surface errors such as misspellings and mistakes in grammar and punctuation to improve what the stories intend to communicate to the actor at first and then to the readership. I removed identifiers such as names or wards and assisted the narrative flow. All names have been altered to anonymise the children and protect their identities. Stories are based on human synergy, communication, motivation and engagement with drama at times of difficulty. In the hope that stories will illustrate applied theatre practice in paediatrics, I am presenting them as an opportunity to engage with what it means to be a child in a hospital reality. Real is relevant, of course. Thus, it becomes almost impossible to accurately define the input of hospital experience in the fictional product in synergistic performance and vice versa. It is a fusion of moments that is not always measurable. There are blends of aromas of joy and drops of sweat and fear that can be sensed and smelled in children's stories, but the meaning of it remains uncaptured and open to interpretation. It does not matter what stories say; they do not have to be ingenious, imaginative and innovative, although I think they are. Despite the length, content and purpose, I honour all stories as precious gifts that children made for us, adults. It is all about how the stories invite us to sense the atmosphere in environments of illness and suffering to help us better understand the personal experience of children and consequently develop great empathy and compassion when working with them. It is here that the stories of this chapter may be of value. I would encourage the reader to be open to observing their sensations and make their meanings while reading the stories. Meaning is personal. I invite the reader to see the stories in this chapter as essential reminders of human strength in times of trouble.

Jane: 'The piano is on fire'

> *It is late at night. A spaceship in the shape of a banana is landing in the park. I can see it from my window. Aliens are coming out of the spaceship. They are four-legged creatures with long, thin arms. They are carrying a piano with them. A princess and a prince are hopping down from the spaceship. The aliens are running back into the spaceship. The princess is playing the piano. She is not bad. The prince is singing. His voice is amazing. Curious monkeys are gathering around the piano. I can see their yellow eyes sparkling in the dark. They play hide and seek, duck, duck, and goose. The princess is upset. 'Stop it!'. The monkeys are running up and down the piano keys. 'Stop it!' The monkeys are eating the piano. 'Go away!' The monkeys want to break the piano. 'Go away!' The monkeys want to burn the piano. 'Get lost! The piano is on fire! I can see the fire. I see the smoke. I hear it crackle. I can feel the heat. 'Get lost!' The monkeys ran at a speed of a rocket! The prince and his princess are crying . . . they are not happy. They want to hide. The moon is out in the sky. 'The moon makes you fly!' says the princess. 'Let's go home', says the prince. The prince and the princess are lifted into the sky.*

In the Burn Unit, we met Jane, an exceptionally imaginative ten-year-old patient. At first, the child was reluctant to participate in the performance. She thought it was more appropriate for younger children and probably less suitable for girls, but she agreed to the bedside entertainment. She must have consented to the project out of boredom and despair, feeling meaningless. She watched the TV for 4 hours because nothing else was there for her to do. Her caregivers confessed that the TV was separating the girl from them.

On the ward, the actor sensed that Jane would benefit from skipping the introduction and cutting away to the most creative part of the project, where the audience is invited to make their own story. The actor and the child explored ideas about travelling in space by rocket, visiting a planet, attending a concert and playing the piano on the moon. While every child is unique, Jane brought her personal experience playing the piano to the performance. They also reflected on Jane's experience dressing up as a princess for school events. Both elements of the child's real life, the piano and the princess, informed the choice to explore the 'princess' character through an aesthetic form familiar to the child, such as playing with a princess Playmobil toy. The child was in a good mood throughout the intervention. She seemed to enjoy playing with her Playmobil set. 'It was as if they were at home', mum said. In addition, the actor facilitated interactive storytelling through puppetry to engage the child in telling her own story in response to the performance. The work was produced spontaneously in direct communication with the child aiming at an organic production of individual stories rather than a critical lens on creativity and communication. Through this kind of participatory synergies, the performance became the beginning and stimulus that engaged the child with a story theme. The gentle and playful dialogue with the child created aesthetic representations of Jane's narrative. Jane was given the role of a detective who watched incidents outside the window. She was asked to imagine that she was capturing people's movements on a video camera. The story-making activity lasted 25 min.

The first time I read Jane's story, I incorrectly assumed that her story reflected a personal incident. Because the prompt-based process involved Jane actively, it seemed that the child was a survivor of a fire accident. I was sure that what made me think of the fire accident was the 'burn ward'. I assumed that the burning piano in Jane's story is a 'by-product' of personal experience. From a scientific perspective, paediatrics burns are the 'forgotten trauma of childhood' (Holland 2006). A burn injury can be a very traumatic experience, not just for the injured child but for the whole family. I guessed that Jane articulated personal memories through aesthetics by engaging with performance, puppetry and objects to devise her own story. Collaborative bedside performance is a process in which children are actively included, as often happens in mediated representations of lived experience (Alrutz 2015). Through a critical reflection of my perceptiveness, I realised that making assumptions about the meaning of stories is complicated. As I read the story several times, I understood that my assumption was a marriage of reading about paediatrics burns and my desire to learn more from the story about the child's emotional needs. I immersed myself in the story, possibly hoping that I could find my way to understanding practice in paediatrics about emotional expression better.

What surprised me in Jane's story is her kindness to the prince and the princess. She lets them escape into a better place far away from the Earth in the end. Is, then, story making in paediatrics escapism? By allowing the escape from the fire, I wonder if the girl was also acting with kindness and generosity. By opening herself to the possibility of *'flying back home'*, she may discover an 'escape' from the hospital in the story through the protagonists. I can only assume this might be a possible reading of the story. If that is the case, although it may only be my speculation, the girl translated core emotions as experiences of liberation and hope. Jane ended the suffering of the characters in a magical way. *'The prince and the princess are lifted into the sky'*. For the characters of her story, the sky was an escape, a break from reality and a better place. She may wish to do for herself, an expression of her need to return to normality. It almost seems that Jane rehearsed her 'escape' in fictional conditions that could potentially imply a wishful preparation for her discharge from the hospital. With no expectations of Jane to use the opportunity to tell a story in specific ways, it is rewarding to see that the child was highly engaged and that telling a story enhanced her confidence to participate in creative activities during her stay in hospital. Jane could have followed a passive role in storytelling by following the existing narrative in the 'Rocket-Arts' performance. Still, she took agency in the performance, playing with Playmobil toys and offering original ideas to redirect the narrative through her story. That is an example of how applied theatre practice in hospitals gives opportunities for children to participate at the level they wish and can do, which is an outcome of adequate encouragement and support and ways of being creative in illness.

Sheila: 'A moon made of cheese'

> *The astronaut looked out of the spaceship to see the moon had turned into cheese. Yummy! The astronaut likes cheese on pasta. She jumped out of the spacecraft, onto the cheese, and dived into the cheese holes. There was a fat mouse. His tummy was full of cheese. 'What are you doing?' the astronaut asked the mouse. 'I have my dinner,' said the mouse. The mouse ate all the cheese he wanted and ran away. A big marshmallow man tried to get the mouse. 'What are you doing' the astronaut asked the big marshmallow man.*
>
> *'I am trying to make me some dinner', said the marshmallow man. The astronaut cut a piece of cheese and offered it to the marshmallow man. He ate all the cheese he wanted and ran away. A monster came to catch the marshmallow man. The beast was hungry and looking for biscuits and sweets. 'What are you doing?' the astronaut asked the beast. 'I have marshmallow with my banana pie', said the monster. The monster had big ears and a big nose but was very skinny. The astronaut cut a piece of cheese and offered it to him. The monster ate all the cheese he wanted and fell asleep. There was enough cheese for everyone on the moon. So after that, the astronaut had a big piece of milky cheese and jumped back into the spaceship to bring her home to Earth.*

Sheila was a lovely seven-year-old girl admitted to the hospital to have surgery. Her operation was scheduled for the afternoon after the bedside performance. Sheila, like many children, was worried before surgery. According to Yang et al. (2022), around 60% of children experience significant anxiety before surgery. These children feel frightened, cry, grasp their loved ones tightly or try to escape. Such behaviours may increase the difficulty in anaesthesia induction, the risk of emergence agitation and even psychological disorders. In Sheila's story, one might assume that there is a hidden feeling of distress and a need to escape. However, as in Jane's story, in reality, we will never find out how much personal detail Sheila infused in her story and if the 'moon made of cheese' directly relied on the child's pre-operative experience.

As the actor visited Sheila, I was watching from a distance looking for different signs of nervousness, movements or visual cues that Sheila might give off, more than likely unknowingly. Children often don't have the language to express their feelings and needs, so paying attention to non-verbal cues is essential to understanding the child's experience. Therefore, there were moments in the first few minutes of the visit when I would pay attention to the use of body language of the actor and the child. However, this was not done for the sake of the performance in its own right, but to understand if the invitation to participate was accepted or rejected by the child. Sheila was nervous at the beginning. The actor bent down to the child's bed level to enable positive non-verbal communication, turned to face the child and used lots of eye contact. Sheila looked away and broke eye contact, which showed nervousness. Then, the actor used his body language to show Sheila that he was trying to understand her feelings. For example, the actor nodded and looked sad because Sheila looked sad. He also used a calm, reassuring tone of voice. He employed a relaxed body posture and facial expression while talking to the child. The actor used a soft and soothing voice while introducing a child-friendly breathing technique to help the child feel calm. Being a relaxed and confident performer is significant to the quality synergy between the actor and the participant child because it sends the message that the actor is ready to listen (Sextou & Hall 2015). Sheila turned her face to her parent and avoided any action with the actor, which was respected. I sensed that the actor was perceived as an unwanted invader in that context. And yet, it can only be assumed that both the child and the actor could find the condition of being in the same space upsetting or hyper-stimulating. However, the way things developed during the performance reveal otherwise.

Sheila's story skips the essential element we might reasonably assume is the actual surgery. She invents aspects of the story that she wants to tell us: to eat all the cheese she wants and run away. Sheila's story is humorous, packed full of funny and creative characters and metaphors, and is probably indicative of her way of dealing with nervousness through her imagination. However, Sheila feels no need to describe her natural anxiety about the pre-operative tests or what she experienced while waiting for her procedure. The repetition of the question 'What are you doing?' and the excitement of eating cheese and running away seems pretty innocuous; they are not saying anything directly about her pre-operative experience. However, we know from the hospital teacher that Sheila showed nervousness about her operation that morning. We also know that the girl was fasting and was only allowed to drink clear liquids a few hours before her surgery.

Surprisingly, the story does not stand as a warning for the parents or the healthcare professionals to attend and manage the child's worries associated with the surgery. It is interesting to note that even though there are many different characters, including a monster, in Sheila's story, the child does not provide any detail about her worries. She says, '*There was enough cheese for everyone on the moon*'. The fact that Sheila speaks of concerns does not mean that worry does not exist, but it may be that the involvement in storytelling made her feel more relaxed. It could, however, be that the tension in the room and some aspects of preparation for the surgery could be more unpleasant than the surgery itself. Allowing Sheila to participate in making the story despite her nervousness at the beginning is not just a lesson of trusting the ability of hospitalised children; it also demonstrates how synergies between the actor and the child provide opportunities to experience exciting moments of creativity during illness. It also reveals how stories enable children to be humorous, resilient and imaginative during struggles.

Most remarkable about Sheila's story is the confidence and energy she developed during the artistic intervention and the unique sense of ownership. The child became more focused on breathing and body sensations as the story came together. While much of the time, in the beginning, was spent on relaxation, the actor also began to introduce the story from early on. Breathing was integrated into the storytelling as a starting point for the 'Rocket-Arts' project. The actor and the child suggested space, stars and galaxies and developed ideas about children travelling in space and becoming great explorers. Neither the actor nor the child could claim the story because they owned it together. Of course, a hospitalised child who experiences pre-operative anxiety cannot articulate a long and coherent narrative. Putting their ideas into a comprehensive shape fell on the hospital teacher, who committed to ensuring that the written story came from the child's involvement.

Paul: 'The naughty Wolf'

> *The Captain spent more time travelling in space than staying on Earth. His mission was to fight space dinosaurs trying to destroy the galaxy. Captain fell off a rock and hurt his head during one of his fights with a two-headed dinosaur. He was bleeding badly. He was terrified. His crew called a space ambulance to take him from Mars back to Earth. The driver of the ambulance was a stupid space wolf. On Earth, they admitted Captain to a hospital where he met Dr Jo. Dr Jo looked after him. Captain was scared. 'What's going to happen to me?' asked Dr Jo. 'Do not worry, it will be alright,' Dr Jo replied. Then, he did a scan of Captain's head. During the scan, the space wolf jumped on Dr Jo and started licking his face. Naughty Wolf! They sent the space wolf back to the spaceship. Captain felt tired in the hospital and asked, 'Please, can I go home?' but Dr Jo said, 'It would be better to stay in hospital and rest." Captain was so sad that he started crying. Dr Jo helped Captain get in bed, and a nurse gave him his medication, but they would not call the ambulance to drive Captain home. Captain fell fast asleep. He dreamt that the space wolves were on the island fighting monsters. Captain saw his nanny during the battle, whom he loved so much. He wanted to say to his nanny, 'Can you take me home?'*

We met Paul, an eight-year-old boy playing with his dinosaur toys in the cardiac ward. Paul was quiet at first but cooperative. The boy animated a Playmobil robot and made his own story. He went to Mars with his dinosaur and the other characters in the story. His mother participated in the story making.

Boy: This is the hospital where I was born (in the story).
Mum: That was a very happy day!
Actor: We have two astronauts and a dinosaur. Where do you want them to go?
Boy: To Mars. Can my mum come too?
Actor: Of course!
Mum: Off we go!

In his play, Paul counted from 10 to 1, and they all took off. One princess, one fairy, one unicorn, three robots, five dogs, three astronauts, one explorer vehicle and his mum held his hand during the activity. They saw stars, aeroplanes, comets and other planets. They landed back on Earth. Throughout the performance, the boy communicated verbally by using simple vocabulary. He made some decisions about his story and created a setting for his spacecraft on Mars. He was creative with toys and imaginative. He particularly liked the robots and animated them with concentration until the end of the activity.

Paul had had the bedside performance the previous week. On that first time he participated in 'Rocket-Arts', the boy decided to go on space adventures as Captain saw a dinosaur with two heads. He returned to Earth to tell his princess about the monster. When the princess finds out, she goes on a space rocket to meet the dinosaur but runs away because the monster is a big bear. She is safe in the space rocket travelling back to Earth. The following week, the boy had 'Rocket-Arts' again and picked up the story from where he had left it. He remembered Captain and the princess. Then he and the princess visited Devon Cliffs together but unfortunately, he fell off one of them. He smashed one eye and was admitted to the hospital. They had an X-ray and were moved onto a ward. The princess and Captain escaped from the hospital. They reached far into the universe and landed on Mars with sand and a beautiful beach. Mum said, 'That was great for him. I am so impressed by how much he enjoyed it after a long meeting with a team of consultants'.

The third time Paul had the project bedside and engaged with the story immediately. The actor skipped the introductory part with the puppets and moved straight to playing with the little people (Playmobil toys) in the space rocket. This time Paul brought Simba, the spaceman and the space robot to help the paramedics to help Jess and take her home. I was impressed by Paul's 'reverse story' that starts from Mars returning to Earth rather than the other way round. One would expect the children to start from a place or event related to their experience (on Earth), but he set their relatable story on a planet away from Earth. And yet, Captain had to be admitted to hospital. It seems that problems and difficulties follow people. They bring them along wherever they go.

Paul's story describes the situation of a boy with a long-life condition who misses normality and how interactive performance helped him express tiredness and feelings of homesickness. Many elements in the story may resonate with any actor or nurse who has worked with children and young people long-term. As we read the story, we could see his almost persistent please, begging, 'Can I go home?' 'Home' as a concept returns. Paul's parents were emotionally moved during the story. The actor knew that dinosaurs were Paul's favourite characters and learned that offering the child an opportunity to use his toys together with Playmobil was a potentially successful way of engaging him in the performance. Fortunately, Paul's acceptance of this offer helped the actor start a one-to-one activity that led to the animation of toys as characters in a non-structured story and improvisatory dialogues. Paul's mother shared feedback with us.

> *The first time he had the spacecraft project, he was very excited. He told all about it to his grandparents. We made planets out of balloons together. We video-tubed rockets, aliens, spaceships, and UFOs. He had many questions about the universe, gravity, stars, and a fundamental question 'how big is space?' So this small project led him to Science and English. You opened a lot of doors for my son. He was so enthusiastic about the project he could not stop talking about it. We talked about stars, life on earth, and life in space. We made artwork and wrote stories. Thank you so much.*

Telling stories did not aim to lead to learning about science but rather to offer opportunities for expression through emotional and social interaction, the possibility of engaging meaningfully in the project. However, providing children with artistic stimuli to create fictional stories and characters by interacting with actors and toys further encouraged this. Paul's mother saw potential in her son's engagement with performance and story making. Still, we cannot be sure how and why the child responded to follow-up discussions and activities in a particular way. Therefore, I make no claims of pedagogical approaches through theatre in this case. Still, I intend to present evidence that supports the educational potential of participatory dramas with puppets in hospitals in Chapter 4.

Alex: 'My grandfather's wellies'

> *Once upon a time, a pair of wellies was in a village shop. They were waiting and waiting for someone to buy them. One day a man went into the shop. He had a long white beard. He pointed to the wellies and said, "Ah, these I like!". He tried them on, and they fit all right. It was autumn, the sun was shining, and it was beautiful. He lived close to the park. There was a lake there. He put on his boots, took his basket and poles, and went to the park. Wellies were happy. The wellies were fishing buddies with the man. One day the man fell from a cliff and couldn't walk. His foot was swollen. It could be broken. "Ah, just what I needed," he said between his teeth. He called for help, and his brother came and carried him home. He couldn't walk and did not go fishing that day. His boots were sad. The next day the man was not well. He stayed in bed. The doctor visited him and ordered, "Stay at home!" His wellies were stuck in his room with him. One day the man died. It was winter. So his boots got angry, and they walked away. "We can go anywhere," they said. They walked on the road, went to the park, and jumped in the snow. They got all muddy! They returned home to dry off. The house was quiet. "Why did you die?"*

This is a story told by Alex, a boy in cardiology who lost his grandfather when he was admitted to a children's hospital for treatment. Danton et al. (2020) argue that children experience a full range of emotions or overreact emotionally after someone in the family dies. Bereaved children may feel separation anxiety and develop behavioural changes such as withdrawing from activities and disturbances in eating or sleeping. Dealing with loss is a very challenging ride for a child. Children can feel lonely, sad, disappointed and wrongly angry with the deceased because something of that relationship remains. Undeniably, the vulnerability of a hospitalised child who is bereaved is quite an extraordinary situation. The child is isolated from their usual support networks, family and friends because of illness. The whole situation in the hospital added to the difficulty of coping with grieving and caused increased anxiety in those children who experienced loss during their hospitalisation. There are, of course, other factors, less tangible, though no less critical, that may cause difficulties for children. These experiences carry with them memories of lived experiences with family and friends. While I focus more on the present time when children live in a hospital, the memories of the child with a loved person represent part of the child's identity. When goodbyes have not been said appropriately, losing part of their identity and the copying process can be even more challenging.

Alex participated in 'Rocket-Arts' with the assistance of a hospital teacher. Although the programme did not refer to or negotiate the loss of a loved one, Alex told the story of an object that belonged to his grandfather. He chose to tell the story of his grandfather's fishing boots a few weeks after he learned about his grandfather's death. The story was developed in a dialogue with the actor and documented by a teacher. Here the story is presented as a narrative rather than a conversation. For example, the actor asked, 'how did the boots feel?' or 'what happened to the old man?' The child replied, 'they were sad' and 'he died'. That was phrased in the story below as '*His boots were sad*' and '*One day the man died*'. The boy's words still keep their freshness and originality by turning into a story: the story of creating, whatever the difficulties, with integrity and excitement.

When I first read Alex's story, an essential question was why he chose to tell a story about fishing boots. His story is disassociated from the performance. Connections, if any, to spaceships, planets and galaxies are not immediately apparent. I will try to answer this question based on Gibson's theory about 'transitional objects' after death. 'In grieving, as in childhood, transitional objects are means of both holding on and letting go' (Gibson 2008, p. 34). Gibson argues that insignificant objects become significant after the owner's death to those who loved the deceased. Clothes can become holders of important memories of those who died and memories of those left behind. In this context, grandfather's wellies were emotionally and symbolically transitional objects; they probably mediated Alex's relationship with his grandfather. Perhaps those wellies held many memories for Alex. Maybe the wellies were one of his grandfather's cherished possessions, thus making them unique to Alex. It is possible that the wellies were part of how Alex's eyes perceived or imagined his grandfather's identity as a competent fisherman. And yet, these are just assumptions, personal interpretations. However, what fascinates me is that Alex claimed these memories in his story. It may be because he could not visit his grandfather anymore. Or maybe Alex was trying to unconsciously create a connection with his grandfather after he was gone by retrieving images of him wearing his wellies on a beautiful sunny autumn afternoon. Or maybe it was just a game of Alex's imagination, a desperate attempt to fill in the space created by his grandfather's death. After some time, these boots could be packed away in Alex's memory and forgotten. But when Alex was in hospital facing his challenges, he possessed those boots and made them his own in his story. This may have allowed him to keep his emotions and control his grief until he became ready to let go.

The emotional space that 'Rocket-Arts' created for Alex to express his grief cannot be overlooked or undervalued. If we assume that the story Alex shared was one of mourning, then his story shows another face, or side, to Alex that our understanding of children in hospitals shows. It is about a child deeply connected to memories of his grandfather, who was deeply angry when his grandfather died. During his hospitalisation, Alex probably had no opportunity other than the storytelling project to give meaning to his emotions and value his loss. Talking about his loss in the story involves the transference of the wellies from the village shop and his grandfather's house to the hospital setting. The image of the wellies in Alex's story is not necessarily realistic or accurate, not necessarily without change, additions of colour or characteristics.

However, Alex chose to tell the story of those wellies and, through them, tell the story of how he heard, thought of or imagined his grandfather's death. The boots might represent his grandfather for the time he is alive in the story. Still, later, during his grandfather's illness and after his death, the boots potentially express the boy and his feelings of sadness and anger, both intense experiences of the bereavement process. Lascaratou (2007, p. 135) argues that it is essential to understand how emotions are conceptualised through metaphorical language. It is the same complexity of putting intense human experiences into literal words to motivate the use of metaphorical language as a resource in understanding illness and communicating it to others. Along these lines, the language of emotions requires attention from adults. That is if adults wish to understand how children feel when they are in hospital and how they process their feelings through the art form. That is why stories allow us to understand how pain is conceived, perceived and even imagined when a child is in hospital. In entering the fictional space during 'Rocket-Arts', Alex becomes, in a way, the owner of his emotions and a user of metaphor for describing a painful situation, something that troubles him and upsets him. Ultimately, by doing that, he gives context to his emotions. Winston's Wish (2020) states in the charter for bereaved children that 'bereaved children are helped by being encouraged to tell the story of what has happened in various ways. These stories need to be heard by those important people in their lives'. I know from experience that grieving tends to create stories of being with the deceased in their imagination. They can consciously or unconsciously make up stories that blend memories with fiction to help the coping process and comfort their hearts. They experience a sense of loss because they no longer have their beloved ones in their lives but carry their memories with them. This is an authentic story that captures how Alex felt at that time. It evidences his need to share his feelings about the loss of his grandfather in a marvellous, poetic, indirect and symbolic way. Thus, I decided to include Alex's story in the book. Nevertheless, how Alex perceived the death of his grandfather and how he remembers him today is uncertain. But there is something in this uncertainty that creates essential possibilities.

Sandy: 'We need the Pancakes'

> Once upon a time, a princess travelled from one place to another and got tired. She wanted to go far away and find a planet. She went on a spacecraft with her friends Lisa and Pippa. She liked going on adventures with them because they were funny. On the blue planet, the princess and her friends were amazed. They got in their Explorer vehicle and found a spot where they started digging. They found big pancakes and put many of those in their school bags. Suddenly, they heard a sound. 'Listen!' the princess said to their friends. 'Did you hear that?' It was a wild white big bear. 'Don't eat us!' The bear bent to see the princess better. Then she spotted their school bags. 'What have you got in there?' she asked them with a threatening voice. 'Pancakes', the princess said. The bear opened her round eyes wide. She was so frightening. 'These pancakes belong to me. Put them back!' The princess took a deep breath and said, 'We need the pancakes. We will send them to children on Earth because they are poor children. The bear asked her, 'where are these places?' and she said, 'Everywhere!' The bear covered her eyes with her hands and stood still. Then, she said 'Fine'. So they attached the pancakes to parachutes and dropped them in places on Earth where poor children live. Some pancakes were dropped in the sea, and the fish ate them.

We met Sandy, a ten-year-old long-term patient with visual impairment. Children with visual impairments rarely take in information unintentionally. Kamei-Hannan (2020) argues that a multi-sensory storytelling approach to listening comprehension and language is a promising intervention for children with visual impairment in increasing their language skills. When performing for children with visual impairment, it is almost impossible to escape the adaptation of the story to fit the needs of those children. For children who are blind or have low vision, the gap left by the visual information can be frustrating. During the performance, the actor talked Sandy through what was happening on the 'stage' – the movement of Playmobil toys and puppets, the props changes, the description of the space rocket's interior and other important visual cues to the performance. This was made possible, thanks to the flexible structure of the performance and the liberty of improvising between scenes, pausing to feed in the information for Sandy, and creating opportunities for interaction between the artist and the child. Although the actor had not rehearsed the story for children with visual impairment, luckily, she was familiar with the audio description service in the main theatre. The service enables people who are blind or have low vision to access the rich elements on offer onstage, helping them be more in the moment and place scenes in context (Andriani 2016). The child knowing the context (adventures in space) and physical detail of the performance (space rocket, toys and puppet descriptions) and having an opportunity to touch objects and play with them throughout the performance made a significant difference to Sandy's experience.

Sandy was one of the most talkative, excited and animated participants we ever had met. He was very interactive with the actor, creative in using toys in his story and quick in making decisions about the characters and the plot. A hospital teacher emphasised the importance of tactual exploration, such as hands-on learning for pupils to purposefully explore objects and puppets, take in information, build concepts and understand how things relate and the world around them. The teacher voiced:

> *It was that boy with vision impairment who perceived puppet Jo well. He asked to touch the puppet, put his fingers in her mouth many times, and joined happily. He has to imagine everything, but it was nice that he was given a chance to visualise what the puppet looked like.*

More specifically, Sandy was agitated in anticipation of what would happen next. When the actor presented a box with Playmobil toys, the teacher led Sandy's hand to touch the box and explore its shape; Sandy couldn't wait for the tube of toys to open. He knocked on the box (knock knock!) and put his ear on it to hear any voices coming from inside. Somehow he guessed that little people were in the box (Playmobil toys). The actor went with his pace to help him calm down. The box was opened, and the actor described the content to Sandy. There was a dog in an ambulance. The child asked, 'What is a dog doing in there?' and laughed. He then asked, 'Can I play with the dog?' and barked like a dog many times. The actor invited the child to make his own story, and he said, 'Me? Can I?' The boy played with the dog and the explorer vehicle for about 5 min and then had the storytelling experience. The boy and the actor with the explorer vehicle during participation discovered blue diamonds. At first, it might seem that there is not too much to learn from Sandy's story. His story is about pancakes and the children who found them and the bear who let them get away with stealing them. However, the emphasis of this story is on how he could 'see' the need for kindness, and his story provides a lesson for all to be generous and giving, be thoughtful and caring for others.

Claire: 'Silence'

'..
....
....'.

Claire was a quiet and reserved child in critical care. Her mother wrote a story to describe their life together:

> *A little girl grew up in a small house in the country. She was the youngest of her siblings. She was much loved, but she often seemed locked in a glasshouse. She could not*

discuss her feelings, so her family tried to understand how she felt through eye contact and the glass. Many times others felt like she was ignoring them. These were horrible moments for them. They had no way to comprehend why. But then, it was impossible. Their emotional dialogue was held back. She loved the attention. She enjoyed affection. Some creative activities were a way of expressing what was kept inside. That little girl could smile. Her smile was a mystery, though. She could focus on puppets and smile during the musical parts. She could look upright when she wanted to communicate happiness and satisfaction. She did that a lot. She was fully aware of what was happening around her, but she needed a 'nudge' to express her thoughts and emotions in her way. Because she didn't speak, it doesn't mean she didn't feel and think! And those who loved her knew that she was enigmatic but exceptional.

We discussed Claire's experience with the hospital teacher. We will never know precisely what Claire thought during the story, but we know that the story stimulated her to communicate with her environment and experience. In particular, the space rocket proved to be a stimulus that activated Claire to remain focused on the performance. Yet, questions about how the child processed the experience will remain unanswered. After talking with the artist about Claire's muted reactions to the performance, I realised that communicating with a child who remains distant from an audience is extremely hard. Part of the artist said, 'I felt challenged by performing to a child with a serious condition', while the other part of her countered with 'I enjoyed being able to give joy'. Instead, she would perform to an audience that responds in ways that she incorporated into her acting with less anxiety about the outcome of participation in the performance. The actor carried an internal self-criticism for feeling bad because she would instead prefer to perform to children who reason with the story and react to her acting as if she was responsible for Claire's situation. The actress did not take responsibility for the child but felt helpless and questioned her acting skills.

I started to think about questions about the artistic process in contexts of silent illness. These questions focus on acting with ill children and provoke further discussions on the actor's role in paediatrics, their thinking and feelings. Some actors, for example, have the desire to make a big difference in children's lives through theatre, to help them become optimistic about their health, to feel better about themselves, to be more creative and imaginative during the performance, but is it possible to achieve such a demanding set of tasks? The interaction between the actor and audience makes them feel better and helpless, seeing them not feeling well. The core feeling held in the actor is the sadness or anger at the sight of children suffering. Sometimes, however, talented actors develop a sense of 'why this child is suffering'. In Claire's case, the actress needed guidance on dealing with the complex and unexpected silence during her performance. She was looking for answers to how to interpret the language of silence. At the same time, she was influential, inventive and focused on her performance. She was the one who paid attention to the bodies moving slowly, attempting a dialogue, an unspoken dialogue between herself and the child. She focused on the rhythm of the breath.

She used her imagination to experiment with silence and tried guessing Claire's invisible wishes. She struggled to find easy ways to challenge the sadness in environments of illness, and she found it difficult to accept the thought that the audience does not gain empowerment and a sense of control over her body. However, she brought Claire's blinking to her awareness and held it as an image or sensation. Other actors performing for critical care children have joined this 'dance' within the silence.

Karim: 'No!'

> There was an astronaut who liked scuba diving. He landed on the moon with his dog named Duffy. They were drilling for gold on the moon but could not find any. They walked up a space mountain, looking for a cave where they could find gold. They went into the cave to explore. It was spectacular! There was a pool full of melting gold. They both took their helmets off, put their heads in gold, and blew golden bubbles. They could see stars made of gold. 'Look up, Duffy! There is a hole on the cave roof,' the astronaut said. Deeper and deeper, they dived into gold, where they found six pieces of gold rocks. 'It's a treasure, Duffy!' Duffy reached out for the gold when suddenly, an ear-piercing alarm went off! An army of treasure guards appeared out of nowhere. They came toward threatening them with their big laser guns. They had been hiding in the darkness. The astronaut screamed, and Duffy hid behind a big rock. The astronaut was so scared; his spacesuit was moist with sweat. Then Duffy said, 'Let's get out of the cave'. But 'oh no! the opening was blocked'. 'Let's dive back into the pool,' said Duffy, but the astronaut replied, 'No, Duffy, we need to get out. Hurry!' From the corner of his eye, he saw a red button on a rock. The astronaut pressed the button, and the stones under their feet started rolling. 'It's an earthquake!' Duffy jumped up on the astronaut's back.

We visited Karim, aged 9, many times throughout the year. He said 'No' to nurses, teachers and actors who offered him activities bedside. Karim was not willing to engage in any conversation with them. Karim would hide under his blanket whenever anyone apart from his parents came to see him, only peeking out occasionally to see what was going on or reach for his phone. The first time we visited Karim, he came across as rude, but we understand that a child in his situation may feel angry about it all. I think the boy was in denial. It was his first day in the hospital, and he did not like it. He did not like anything we offered him. So we sang a song and interacted on his terms. He said, 'I don't like puppets; I don't like toys'. Over time, Karim would refuse to sing more songs with the puppet, although he would giggle at the story. He recognised colours from the space rocket and made paintings of planets from various story scenes. However, his response to every invitation by the actor to make his own story was 'no!'

When a nurse came and disconnected him from the machine, he darted off to run up and down the ward after being cooped up in bed for a long. He spotted the portable space rocket set entering the ward at that time. He enthusiastically returned to his bed and listened to the story with the other patient and his mum. He participated with joy and laughter and had many suggestions for Simba for flying his rocket to space. Afterwards, he made objects and characters out of clay. His

46 Sick children's stories

teacher commented that that was the longest time he had interacted with anyone in one session. However, his response to invitations to make his own story was a big non-negotiable 'no!'

In entering Karim's bedside space – the sphere of personal space and identity – professionals shift their role as nurses, teachers or actors in a subjective way; that is how the child regards them in bed. Professionals become the 'other', the 'unfamiliar adult', the 'stranger' amongst other strangers on the hospital ward, visiting the child during the day for various reasons. They often lose their ability to be friendly or trusted, not because they are so but because the child sees no appeal in them visiting the bedside. There is something in this movement of roles from the hospital space to the private sphere, from public acceptance to personal intolerance, that makes meaningful connections to Karim's story. One day, he rejected all opportunities for creative play and story making again until the moment the actor gave him a Playmobil astronaut set. Once he got possession of his toy, he became engaged. He wanted to skip the introduction with the puppets and go straight to the story to use his astronaut. His appetite to participate in the report may have developed because he felt essential to it, someone who could have control over his toy, control over his performance and extended control over his illness. It may also be that he wanted his mum happy. His mum was worried about him, but the boy told her to 'Be brave' to make her feel better. We were thrilled to witness this moment as it was special. On another day, Karim listened to the story but remained silent while lying in bed. He would only speak with a whisper when invited to engage, but he unexpectedly started coming out of his shell when engaging with the story he knew well. He smiled at the actor and played as usual. She tried to keep him relaxed in anticipation of his surgery. The actor asked Karim once more if he were in the mood to make a story for Simba, and this time, to everyone's surprise, he said 'yes!'

Lisa: 'A robot who could not dance'

> There was a silver robot living on a rocky blue planet. The robot took pictures of the blue planet. Then, the robot climbed up the ladder of his spaceship, looking for other robots. There were no other robots on the planet. Then the robot played football. It is no fun to play football alone. Then, the robot played a song. And then another one. And then another one. The robot could not dance and be bored and sad. The robot climbed up the ladder of his spaceship again, looking for other robots to play together. There were no other robots around. But, suddenly, a flying robot landed right next to the spacecraft. The flying robot played a song and started dancing. The silver robot was sad. "I cannot dance," said the flying robot. "I will teach you to dance," said the flying robot and played the song again. The two robots danced together. Step, step, step, step. 1, 2, 3, 4. Forward, back, on. One arm up, one arm down. One leg up, one leg down. Twist to the right. Twist to the left. Step, step, step, step. 1, 2, 3, 4. The two robots danced and danced for many hours. That was fun. The silver robot was happy.

We met Lisa and her little brother at the hospital. Lisa was a long-term patient in the dialysis ward. At first, Lisa was unwilling to recognise any Playmobil toys in the portable rocket we used as props in our performance. She did not name those items and made no connections between the story, the toys or rocket. She was either not interested in the story of resisting engaging or had difficulty imagining space and stars as they were not physically present in the room. However, she looked at the rocket for a few seconds and then moved her attention down to the floor and back to the rocket for a while. This sequence happened many times. To make a positive difference in this child's experience, the actor decided to support her in making connections between the story's characters. The hospital teacher agreed to give the child a pack with a brand-new astronaut set and a robot, encouraging her to use it during the performance. The child dropped the astronaut on the floor, but she kept the robot and practised with it with assistance from the hospital teacher.

We performed for that child a month later. We observed that the child used her robot to interact physically with Puppet Jo and started making a connection with the puppet. She smiled at Jo and reached out to touch their hair. She was clapping her hands when Jo was singing and pointing at the rocket when Jo asked questions about how to get travelling. After a few months, we observed more improvements. For example, Lisa recognised the toys in the rocket, and she would sing along with the Puppet Jo. She would even dance on the bed with excitement. To everyone's surprise, that child who did not speak and recognise anything from the story now gave simple commands to the robot 'go', 'up', 'down'. She livened up. She was counting stars (millions!). She played with an astronaut toy, landed him on the moon with his dog Duffy and started drilling for gold. They walked up on a space mountain in her play, looking for a space cave where they found many other alien doggies. They also found six pieces of gold, 'a treasure!' They stayed on the moon because they liked it there. The child seemed to enjoy the toys and play with her brother. 'It was as if they were at home', mum said. According to her hospital teacher, by the end of the school year, the child had made progress in concentration by playing with her robot; she could recognise objects, communicate with the teacher through play and interact with the robot miniature. The teacher followed up the 'Rocket-Arts' story with Lisa. She gradually became more willing to work with her teacher and recreate different story versions, which the teacher described as 'creative distractions' and 'enjoyable activities' during the blood infusion. The child's mother said she was impressed by the child's improvement over time.

Melissa: 'The Planetary'

The astronaut looked out of the window of his spaceship to see the Moon had changed colour. It was black. 'That's strange!' So he got off the spaceship to look at himself and see what was happening. The sky was empty of stars. So he did not know what to do. He went back to his spaceship to call Andy, his friend on Earth and tell him about the Moon changing colour. Bryan, his best friend, said that the Moon changes colours when it changes moods. The astronaut looked at the Moon again. The Moon was a black hole because there were no stars. He had an idea. He makes paper stars, paints them yellow, and makes them float; the sky is full of them. The Moon turned from black to yellow. But the stars ran out of float and fell off the sky. The sky is empty. So the Moon realised the stars were fake and turned from yellow to red. The astronaut was waiting to see if the

> Moon would change colour. Why is the sky empty? Where did the real stars go? Will they come back? The real stars appeared. They only went to bed because it was morning. The astronaut got into his spaceship to fly back to Earth. The moon is like a giant lightbulb.

On the first day we visited Melissa in oncology; she was very poorly, lazy and tired. Procedures and treatment cause pain; therefore, the literature discusses 'painful procedures' and powerful pain memories and the importance of pain management in paediatrics (Carter & Simons 2014). Previous experiences of hospitalisation, treatment, suffering and the consequences of being a long-term patient in oncology can shape how a child frames pain based on expertise (Kortesluoma et al. 2009). Melissa kept asking for her dad, who had gone to get some coffee for him and ice cream for Melissa. She responded verbally to the actor and was interested in the space rocket but did not react physically. The girl picked up the astronaut with the robot Playmobil toy to lead the action. Limited one-to-one interaction was evident during the performance. Although the child did not engage with the puppets at first, when the space rocket came into her cubicle, she became interested in the space rocket, but her concentration was limited. She asked questions about the robot and pushed a button on the toy to make him fly. Despite her lazy mood, the child engaged with the actor and communicated verbally using complete sentences. She soon fell asleep. A week later, we visited Melissa gain. Her spirits were lifted, and her concentration was better this time. The actress, the girl and her mother participated in the performance.

Melissa's story is mixed in how a range of emotions is communicated. This may reflect the broader experience of various emotions related to the assessment and the management of persistent pain during her treatment in oncology. Melissa's story demonstrates the need for the child to face illness in the protection of metaphor. Lascaratou (2007, p. 135) argues that it is essential to understand how emotions are conceptualised through metaphorical language. It is the same complexity of putting intense human experiences into literal words to motivate the use of metaphorical language as a resource in understanding illness and communicating it to others. Along these lines, I think that besides attending to a child's verbal and facial expressions during a participatory performance in a hospital, emotional language also requires attention if we wish to understand better how children feel and how they process their feelings through the art form.

Melissa's story triggered my curiosity. It made me wonder if the story revealed her skill in expressing emotions through metaphor instead of putting her feelings into words. I wonder, is this story about the different phases and colours of the moon? Are the moon's colours a metaphor for the tension between feelings of sadness, worries, loneliness, emptiness, hope and anger and the process of assimilation, adaptation and accommodation of those feelings? On first reading it, I felt that the theme is not the space adventures *per se* but the act of looking at the world (her ill self?) from a distance to Earth – observing herself from outside her emotional experience almost, with eyes open to the changes in her moods and feelings. In this assumption, the moon becomes a metaphor for the purpose the bedside performance tries to fulfil – a tool to help both the child and the performer see with fresh eyes and express emotions, facilitating the synergy between the audience and the actor. Alternatively, I could read the story simply for its content, but stories can be complicated, like theatrical scenes, 'coloured by its intricate entanglement with human desire and fallibility' (Jackson 2007, p. 112).

As I reread the story, I started seeing what colours Melissa sees because that is where the story's focus lies. But, while such a demonstration of illumination is pivotal to Melissa's communication with the artist, it may describe emotions, possibly pain, through emotional language by using colours. Could the story be an indication of observing her pain escalating from sadness (black) to happiness (yellow) and from joy to anger (red)? In my imagination, I could almost see the child trying to 'fix' the problem that is pain caused by chemical treatments such as chemotherapy and radiation by substituting the real stars with fake ones. I continue wondering if Melissa is trying to replace the lack of normality in her life with some kind of 'normality', but despite her best efforts failing to manage her pain because pain overpowers her. Was she trying to retouch and restore her body image that has been affected by treatment by using sparkling stars? Did she manage to repair her ill appearance (and identity) with something beautiful and glittering? I am consciously and deliberately refusing to answer any of the above questions because I think that what matters is not to interpret Melissa's intentions. It is entirely possible that Melissa told us a story about stars inspired by a bedtime story she read the previous night or by watching out of the window during the night when the hospital ward is quiet. However, I believe that one can find meaning in metaphor by searching for clues and patterns in a story and then using them as signs to understand better how participatory performance encourages a child under treatment to communicate pain. This is a partial way of sensing the stories children like Melissa tell in paediatrics and connecting with them in inconsistent but loving ways.

Margaret: 'A park for the animals'

> *The dog and the princess went on space adventures together. Princess (name of the girl) landed on a 'jungle' planet with many animals and dinosaurs. They met with a rainbow and went on a safari. They explored the jungle, where they met a rabbit, a kitty, farm animals, and wild animals. There was a unicorn too. Then, they flew to another planet where they built a park for the animals. Animals were flying out in space. They walked to the park on the new planet and had a party. They all lived happily together with the princess and the dog.*

We met Margaret, a lively and chatty eight-year-old, in the Waterfall ward (oncology). She responded very well to the performance verbally and physically by playing with the little people in the rocket. The girl picked up the princess with the dog Playmobil toy to lead the action. Lengthy one-to-one interaction was evident during the performance. When the actor packed to depart, the girl said to her, 'See you again!' Margaret had a visit from a consultant during the artistic work. When the doctor arrived, the performance was extended to her and became a social event with a doctor–patient communication outcome. The actor stepped back during the examination as she should, but something extraordinary happened. The performance was adapted to change but not discontinued because of the disturbance. That is rare. The girl maintained the fictional context of space and time alone without any help from the actor. The girl preserved the 'fictional bubble', as described in Chapter 1, in which she pretended to be a princess with her dog, looking after space animals and being strong for them. She continued acting out her character as she did before the doctor arrived, and together they engaged in a dialogue that developed organically in fiction within a clinical setting.

Consultant: What is this rocket doing in our hospital?
Girl: It's for the princess and her dog.
Consultant: Am I allowed to see what is inside?
Girl: Yes. Look!
She opened the space rocket's door for the doctor and explained what those animals were doing there. Then, she re-enacted the story by using her toys. The doctor examined her tummy and continued telling the story while she was concerned.
Consultant: And how is the princess feeling?
Girl: OK. A bit tired.
Gonsultant: Does she want to sleep?
Girl: No, she can't. She is looking after her dog and all the animals.
Consultant: I see some astronauts and robots in the space rocket. Can she get them to help her?
Girl: No, they can't. They have to go, you see . . . [and continued with more details about the park and all the exotic birds, the thousands of space animals, etc.].

The medical examination went very smoothly. The consultant thanked her, said goodbye to the princess and moved on to the next patient. After that, a couple of nurses arrived and conversed with the girl about the rocket and the story. The girl told the story again and showed them the rocket's interior. It was all about the princess (the girl had identified herself) and their wonders in space.

There are no neutral eyes to see an incident in the hospital. In my eyes, Margaret took ownership of the story naturally, as a child would typically do in their play. She not only adapted to the new situation of having a clinical examination in the middle of the performance but to everyone's surprise, she invited the consultant to her fictional space by immersing her in her story. It was interesting to see a shift in power between the patient as a passive child and an imaginative, playful child in times of serious illness. The patient earned control over the patient–doctor relationship by controlling the 'as if' situation in which the doctor was immersed. What a contradiction to the norm! The passive child-patient became an active, creative, playful child. This complex exchange can further inform the analysis of the relationship between applied theatre and the practice encountered in non-theatre venues and spaces. No neutral containers exist into which applied theatre is placed as cultural exchanges of power offer valuable frameworks for critical engagement (Thompson 2005). There are tensions between the artistic and clinical culture, fictional and clinical spaces, and concerns about the application of theatre in areas designed for a different purpose rather than storytelling and theatrical improvisation. To the clinician's eyes, the space rocket confuses the sense and focus of the hospital space. It is hard to conceive the intention of bedside performance in a hospital ward. However, play specialists and actors-in-healthcare offer many creative activities to children in hospitals. By highlighting how the consultant responded to the girl's invitation to step into the fiction, a greater understanding of the acceptance of applied theatre practice and the possibilities for clinical staff's engagement with stories can be realised.

We revisited Margaret on the ward two weeks later and found her with her father. She was feeling angry, aggressive and moody. One-to-one interaction took place during the performance. Although she was not seeing it for the first time, the girl was attracted by the rocket and wanted to skip the introduction with the puppets and go straight to the story with Playmobil toys. She was rude, but we understand that a child in this situation may feel angry about life. She was on a new medication, and her body didn't like it. Margaret was a different child on that day. She did not like anything we offered her. She said, 'I don't like puppets'. 'I don't like toys. It is humiliating'. 'I don't want to make a story'. She rejected all opportunities for creative play until the moment the actor gave her a new Playmobil set of a princess with her dog. Once she got possession of HER toy, she engaged and asked her father to bring the princess she had kept from the performance two weeks ago. Now she had two princesses and two dogs, and she picked up the dog to lead the action. She used a range of vocabulary and made many decisions for her story. The child interacted with the actor verbally and developed a short dialogue with her dad.

Child: 'I can see a shadow in the rocket. And there is a diamond. Are there diamonds on the moon? Dad, can you google it?'
Dad: 'Will do'.
Actor: 'Anything can happen in a story'.
Child: 'I will make a story about scuba diving'.
Actor: Scuba diving in space?
Child: 'I will keep the helmet on'.
Dad: Do you think there are lots of diamonds in the sea?
Child: 'I found my first one!'

Melissa responded to the actor's questions, but her responses were slow, and she was physically tired. While the child went to rest, the actor had an informant chat with the child's father about the project and Melissa's remarkable ability to imagine places and make up stories. Her father gave the actor some feedback.

> This project is spot on! It makes us feel so much better. I am emotional now because it has been a long time since the last time someone spent time with my little girl to understand how we feel.

In my view, what Melissa's father describes occurs partly because the focus of the artist is on spending quality time with the child in a performance, which can be reassuring to families about being treated with care and respect, and partly because parents/carers need the reassurance of support and personal attention to cope with their worries. In other cases, when the performance is rushed due to clinical emergencies and diagnostic tests, the actor and the child are distracted by what is happening around them, and the quality of the connection can be compromised. Of course, clinical procedures are prioritised in hospitals, but such interruptions make performance more difficult because the relationship between the artist and the child is broken, and the reassurance for the parents/carers about getting attention to how they feel is dismissed. Luckily, the performance with Melissa ran smoothly with no distractions and time constraints affecting the impact of the work on the child and her father.

Stories of hospitalisation on a stitched land

Let's use a metaphor and suppose that the stories I presented in this chapter are crafted on a 'stitched land' between reality and fiction. Pieces of cloth symbolise lands. Presume we accept that the child as a patient lives in the land of illness (hospital) where they experience unpleasant circumstances (hospital life). The dramatic context introduces a new fictional land (fantasyland) to the child where illness and suffering disappear. In that case, the child is invited as an audience to live between the two lands during the participatory performance, the concept of *metaxis*. In this metaphor, I put the responsibility on the actor. The actor's role is instrumental in securing the two pieces of cloth together with a few stitches, mending tears and restoring the gap between the real and the believed *as if* it is real. Narratives, puppetry, props, films, objects and toys become the threads sewn-in cloth with the gentle movement of the actor in-between real and non-real. The stitched land allows the child to be aware of reality while stepping into a fictional space and time. The actor must secure the stitches to maintain the conditions of fiction. Children can be who they want to be or become on the stitched land. That is how I understand the adoption of new identities in illness through theatre and how I think this chapter's stories gained presence. Performances and stories cannot create accurate copies of 'normal' reality. Still, they can provide a safe and positive environment for a relaxing and reassuring experience. In all honesty, illness and wellness do not matter on the stitched land. The stories actors told to children and the stories children returned were created in a zone out of the ordinary. What matters is having the liberty to stand on the stitches and survive on new land. The stories I presented as examples of my practice are products of this *act of balancing* on the margins of illness and wellness without fear within the safe conditions of drama, possibly evidence of a new 'normality'. It is a great privilege to access these stories because they allow us to build on the work happening in paediatrics in context and with purpose.

The stories children shared also demonstrate an unmistakable sense of enjoyment in the creative ways children use the clinical space during the artistic work, in contrast to their suffering during illness. While it is perhaps to be expected that hospitals are places that evoke negative responses from children associated with clinical stressors (Pelander & Leino-Kilpi 2010), what is less expected is that children can still be playful, creative and imaginative during challenging situations. Hospitalised children in high-risk wards such as Intensive Care Units and Oncology often lose the sense of who they are and their sense of security (Carter & Simons 2014). Despite hospital staff's efforts to humanise the clinical environment, children find hospitals places of painful experience. They want to remove themselves from a frightening place, but they are limited by what they can do to escape. Usually, all they can do is resist cooperating with nurses or turn their heads away from adults and hide under their duvet. At its best, applied theatre practice can make a positive difference in children's experience in medical-dominated environments when it is created with sensitivity and attention to children's needs, abilities and reactions.

In this chapter, I tried to show that applied theatre can make a risk-free environment and provide children with opportunities to use language more confidently, speak and write, and communicate with others. In that sense, the hospital space is transformed into a creative place and the hospital experience is a little more bearable. The stories shed light on how a hospital ward culture can facilitate children's possibilities to feel secure enough to cooperate with an actor, open up, tell stories and communicate through the arts. It shows that intimate performance maintains their self-identity as playful and lively story-makers despite the clinical place's constraints, even in the most challenging moments. The stories are owned by the children who told them. In the same way that Lascaratou (2007) and Scarry (1985) believe that pain exists even when patients are silent, and pain remains 'unspeakable', I would argue that many elements of the hospital experience, including impressions, feelings and emotions, exist even when children keep them hidden and unexpressed. The stories hospitalised children told may show that they had opportunities to speak the unspoken within time and personal ability limits.

The stories prove that participatory practice can curve time and space for children to express emotions safely in the fictional frame. By 'safe', I do not intend to discuss trauma or propose drama as therapy. Performances aimed to engage the children with imaginary worlds that did not refer to or deal with trauma stories. Remarkably, some stories involved emotional content and possible links to children's experiences. Often emotions emerge directly. In Lisa's story, for example, the silver robot was sad and then happy. In Paul's story, the Captain was scared and so sad that he started crying. And in Jane's story, the prince and the princess were crying because they were not happy. In Margaret's story, they all lived happily together. In Karim's story, the astronaut was scared, and in Alex's story, the wellies were happy at first, but when the man died, the wellies were angry and ran away. Other children seem to have tried to express emotions indirectly, subject to personal interpretation. Did Sheila, for example, try to use a language of emotions through the changes of colours of the moon? Did Sandy use a frightening bear to communicate his fear? And were Jane's repetitive orders to the monkeys to 'Stop it!' and 'Go away!' telling us something about her worries? Home is also a recurring theme in the stories of this chapter. I wonder what does home symbolise and communicates indirectly. Is home a theme that describes or explores belonging and not belonging and those that might help children cope with their illness? Jane, Paul and Sheila's stories show the same desire to return home. Was Jane observing difficult incidents from an aesthetic distance, possibly resolving complex incidents in fiction and expressing emotional needs? Carel (2013), philosopher of medicine, argues that 'illness produces a distancing effect, which allows us to observe normal human behaviour and cognition via their pathological counterpart'. But we cannot be sure. There is no clarity on the meaning of 'home', what it might mean for each child and what childhood experiences were attached to 'home' (Wheatley & Baker 2007). The work, in that sense, offered experiences with an appropriate balance of challenges relating to understanding emotions and protection provided by the fictional context.

In the stories of this chapter, children put a subjective value on their emotions; that is how they represent their experiences and feelings. For one reason or another, and I know that this sounds a little vague, the fictional safety children experienced in the storytelling performance liberated them. Children could be completely unaware of how the imaginary conditions help them experience moments of difficulty or pleasure as they go about stories. Alex's story, for example, made me think more deeply about children's emotions when in hospital and enabled a keener understanding of children's experiences of grief. I realised that children have a lot to say and hide when they experience pain, physical or emotional. Yet children do not give much away until someone offers them a window of opportunity to articulate their own stories. We will never know how much personal detail children infuse in their stories and if stories like Jane's directly rely on their experiences. My gut response raises the question of when we should dismiss our conceptions of illness and how should we respond to hospitalised children's circumstances from a neutral position? The challenge is that while I can debate ethics in applied theatre performance in hospitals, I cannot ignore the complexity of managing responses to artistic practice in acute clinical settings. The associated messages of pain and distress in medical places will inevitably be cited in personal understandings and vice versa. One needs to manage their responses to children's experiences in paediatric experiences rather than trusting their knowledge.

Despite knowing that stories are fictional products of the child's imagination, there seem to be emotional-revealing elements in those stories that mean something about the child that requires individual attention and approach. I believe that connections between the audience and the actor created layers of opportunities for expressing an emotional vocabulary by children who found inspiration in the performance. The clinical practice could not be dependent on the work that an actor, of course, facilitates. Still, it may be that better clinical practice becomes available to children because of the actor. By 'better', I mean with intelligent compassion. The stories I presented indicate that communicating through aesthetics in a skilled performative way and being present with the child in the fictional context enables children to use their emotional lexicon even when experiencing pain.

> Even when suffering, people in pain are often highly creative in expressing their suffering – sometimes in words, other times in images and art, and

other times in gestures, ritual utterances, symbols, posture, and performance. By paying careful attention to the languages of pain, medical professionals and patients alike can cooperate more successfully in the healing process. These languages of pain open up a world of meaning, informing us of how people in the past, and today, experience their suffering.

(Bourke 2012, p. 2421)

Having considered Bourke's (2012) view on the languages of pain, I am mindful to avoid extreme claims about applied theatre's powers to provoke impressive results in complicated settings. Many factors may influence a child's expressivity, such as clinical stressors, lack of privacy and normality, separation of significant others, medical treatment and physical pain (Crane 2009). The most frightening is the fear of prospective surgery, causing perioperative anxiety (Fortier & Kain 2015). However, it makes sense to suggest that participatory bedside performance evolves in constant interaction with the determining factors of medical environments. Although the performance can be short, the practice can carve spaces for self-expression and transform the constraints of clinical settings into beautiful, pain-free imagined worlds beyond the time of intimate participation in drama. The stories children told us can evidence that. In acknowledgement of theatre's plasticity to adapt, or resist, in non-theatrical settings, theatre in hospital is a product of negotiation between the artistic and the clinical. The ways stories are told and retold evolve organically in dialogue with the environment led by the synergistic communication between the child and the actor. We need to remember that stories can mean and not mean things. When the impulse comes to read the meaning of a story, awareness of location, perception and interpretation needs to come into play. We must attend not simply to what children produce but also to how we engage with the meaning of those productions. The stories in this chapter may have nothing to say to some people, which is understandable. But to me, these are stories of meaning that one can find in patience and humility because only with patience and humility one can sense how the participant feels.

The stories of this chapter reveal that children move from 'being ill and unable' to the identity of 'being ill and able to tell stories'. This is a process of restoring agency for the patient in healthcare contexts caused by a reallocation of the focus from illness to creative activities, paying respect to the child as a human being (Sextou 2016; Wilson 2022). Through participation in performance, attention is shifted from the negative images of the ill body in 'the kingdom of illness' (Carel 2013) to more positive images of friendly puppets, familiar toys and amusing characters in fantasyland contexts. There seems to be a negotiation of power and a repairing of roles enabled by a comforting and relaxed approach to participatory performance in the hospital. Performance is not seen as something 'fixed and loud' but as a flexible and evolving experience between the actor and the child and an attentive approach to the child's emotional needs rather than a controlled and oppressive one. 'Fixed' here is not defined by the length of time but as a process that blocks interaction, compassion and kindness channels. 'Loud' does not necessarily mean boisterous but lively and intense, which may also cause an anxious or empathetic child further distress and tears during the performance. The actor avoids any ambition to showcase their acting and singing skills but places value on the child's condition and the performance context. By doing that, actors enable the participants to be who they are and express how they feel at that time in opposition to the culture of actors who enter hospital wards to make an impression. This approach challenges the expectation of children to be treated as patients and its associated risks of power and empowerment over the hospitalised child.

I need to clarify that I use the word 'empowering' with caution and give it the meaning of awareness and awakening consciousness. I resist using clichéd expressions such as 'applied theatre is empowering'. The empowering role of applied theatre is rooted in Augusto Boal's Theatre of the Oppressed (1979) and was exhausted by the Theatre for Development practitioners in the 1990s. Theatre in paediatrics is a political action of power per se in many ways. Therefore, I see no need to declare, but I can share my experience and what I witnessed over the years of my hospital practice. I noticed actors finding the power within themselves to be courageous to enter medical places of pain and fear. Control was not imposed on those actors but instead discovered or rediscovered by themselves, driven by a desire to connect with children in difficulty through the art form. I have been privileged to work with many of them and learn from their talents, bravery and professionalism. I also witnessed children finding the power and strength in illness. These children naturally detached from the patient's role and regained their active and creative selves through theatre. Furthermore, it would be wrong to say that applied theatre empowers children to escape the patient's identity because it aims for the opposite. Applied theatre deals with illness conditions in clinical settings and should acknowledge the child's right to be ill, scared, angry, aggressive, anxious and emotional. And yet, I don't mean that the actor gives the child permission to be sick or who they want to be during the performance. Instead, the actor respects the child's psychological and behavioural difficulties and the tensions associated with hospitalisation.

Occasionally, one can witness exciting conversations between actors, children and medical staff, as evidenced in Margaret's story. Such moments make actors jump from their seats with joy and fulfilment, feeling happy for the child and rewarded. But, children usually are not in the mood to interact and communicate when they feel unwell. Some children missed out on parts of the performance either because the artist decided to skip the introduction and go straight into the storytelling because emergencies happen, children had to go for tests, or simply because children fell asleep under the effects of strong medication. These children were not allowed to regain the missing part of the experience unless they were long-term patients, for whom there were opportunities to have the performance bedside again on a different day. However, I have witnessed committed actors engaging children in work, and by watching those children during the performance, we will be surprised by the effort they both, actor and child, make to engage with fiction. Children adopt different identities, attitudes and roles when they are hospitalised. It is impossible to overstate the profound forces of the 'ill person' identity or how strong the culture of being 'unwell' is. I believe that paediatric patients belong to a compassionate clinical culture and a 'vulnerable' identity inherent in their clinical state. I also believe that children in hospitals have adopted the patient's identity and can be good at this, but it does not mean that they like it. It often feels that children wait for a window of opportunity to 'betray' their identity as ill children, step out of their role as patients and reveal their natural talent of being playful, active and interactive as much as their condition allows them. Children's ability to be spontaneous and engage with fiction makes applied theatre in paediatrics possible. Children's stories, in this sense, are signs of commitment, liberation and redefinition.

I have tried to demonstrate the benefits of bedside participatory theatre in enabling communications between the actor and the child with an identifiable impact. Intimate performance offers the participant opportunities to develop a personal narrative reflecting how they understand their world, imagine it, or feature or exist in it. Children can benefit from the opportunity for synergistic exchanges of body gestures, words, ideas and emotions through interactive play may produce complementary information that can be helpful to healthcare professionals. The hidden anger and fear that some stories uncover, such as Jenny, Alex and Sandy's stories, may express power rather than defeat. According to McCormick, some stories reveal the 'unseen process' and how the child finds the words to express feelings that usually people try to avoid; they neglect, reject, ignore and overlook (McCormicK 2012). Spending time finding the phrases, feeling them and using them can be challenging. However, because stories work at a fictional level, they let the child's unconscious inform us how to address their feelings and describe them as they would in their pretend play. Playing with toys and puppets certainly must have enabled this process. Stories continue as extensions of the children that may, or may not, give us an entry into the child's emotional life during hospitalisation. I cannot stop thinking that there are children in hospitals who lack communication skills and that it must have been frustrating for them to want to tell stories but feel restricted by language. This problem needs to be addressed at a macro-level in planning future projects.

Parents occasionally witnessed stories such as in Paul, Sandy, Claire and Margaret's cases. For example, the work we offered to Paul extended the parent's opportunity to interact with their children and enhanced the parent and child's ability to employ the performance experience in other related activities. Thanks to the storytelling, Margaret's father felt reassured by getting involved in the performance and feeling reconnected with his girl. On other occasions, the parental model of support and guidance dominated the child's choices of playing with toys during the performance, which is an essential topic for another discussion. But, what is necessary is the role of applied theatre practice in enhancing connectivity and responsivity and creating opportunities to build or further improve parental relationships with their sick children. I discussed the safe conditions of drama earlier in this book. By reflecting on the stories where parents were either involved or gave feedback to the artist, I refer to applied theatre as a 'safe zone' for parents and children to connect, play and learn together during hospitalisation. Applied theatre practice offered space and time, stimulus and openings for parents/carers and children time and time to interact with each other, redirecting their attention from the child's health condition to other more pleasant topics of discussion than illness. Children and families exercised agency.

Parental integration into the project, primarily through working on educational activities, makes me wonder if applied theatre could be a strategy for engaging parents in delivering quality child healthcare more systematically. According to the Medway NHS Foundation Report (2020/21), the National Health System of England supports the person-focused delivery of care where patients, caregivers and families are listened to and supported by hospital staff to meet their needs. Meaningful engagement is developed through working with children-patients, parent/carer(s) and hospital staff. In Paul's case, it is promising to see that some parents, not all of them, not just appreciate the value of applied theatre in paediatrics but can also extend the theatrical experience by developing new activities with a critical mind. This realisation provides an excellent opportunity to set up dedicated stakeholder advisory groups at the hospital and involve parents and children in co-production. Parents can be the artist's critical friends throughout the projects who would review the aims, develop the tools and materials and advise on ethical audience participation and the content of stories, methods and implementation. Paul's mother would be an excellent advisor working with actors, hospital teachers and healthcare professionals willing to explore what might be achieved by applying theatre and participatory dramas in hospitals. Without art departments and schools in many hospitals worldwide, involving parents in applied theatre practice could be an effective strategy to support children and the arts in healthcare.

In acknowledgement of the complexity of hospitalisation, the emotions enacted within the stories cannot be fully understood in light of the little we know about the children's personalities, life experiences and health conditions. It may be that applied theatre is a means by which the actor inspires and motivates the child to explore possible plots. Correctly decrypting these plots could indicate the enigmatic aspects of hospitalised children's lives. Thus, stories as synergistic products of theatre in paediatrics are unique communications. It is a surprising conclusion; applied theatre enhances our understanding of the child, for theatre generates stories as extensions of children's life that happens on a stitched land between fiction and reality in a hospital.

References

Alrutz, M 2015, *Digital Storytelling, Applied Theatre, & Youth Performing Possibility*, Routledge: London.
Andriani, R 2016, I love theatre, and I'm blind. Here's how that works. *Sydney Festival*. www.theguardian.com/stage/2016/sep/10/i-love-theatre-and-im-blind-heres-how-that-works.
Boal, A 1979, *Theatre of the Oppressed*, Pluto: London.
Bourke, J 2012, 'Languages of pain', *Lancet*, vol. 30, no. 379, p. 9835. https://pubmed.ncbi.nlm.nih.gov/22764375/.
Boyd, B 2009, *On the Origin of Stories. Evolution, Cognition and Fiction*, The Belknap Press of Harvard University: Cambridge, MA.
Carel, HH 2013, 'Illness, phenomenology, and philosophical method', *Theoretical Medicine and Bioethics*, vol. 34, no. 4. https://doi.org/10.1007/s11017-013-9265-1.

Carter, B & Simons, J 2014, *Stories of Children's Pain: Linking Evidence to Practice*, SAGE: London.
Crane, R 2009, *Mindfulness-based Cognitive Therapy*, Routledge: London.
Danton, L, Rapa, E & Stein, A 2020, 'Protecting the psychological health of children through effective communication about COVID-19', *The Lancet Child and Adolescent Health*, vol. 4, no. 5. www.ncbi.nlm.nih.gov/pmc/articles/PMC7270522/.
Fortier, MA & Kain, ZN 2015, 'Treating perioperative anxiety and pain in children: A tailored and innovative approach', *Paediatric Anaesthesia*, vol. 25, no. 1. https://doi/10.1111/pan.12546.
Gibson, M 2008, *Objects of the Dead. Mourning and Memory in Everyday Life*, Melbourne University Press: Victoria.
Holland, AJ 2006, 'Pediatric burns: The forgotten trauma of childhood'. *Canadian Journal of Surgery*, vol. 49, no. 4. https://pubmed.ncbi.nlm.nih.gov/16948886/.
Jackson, A 2007, *Theatre, Education and the Making of Meanings, Art or Instrument?*, Manchester University Press: Manchester.
Kamei-Hannan, C, McCarthy, T, D'Andrea, FM & Holbrook, MC 2020, 'Investigating the efficacy of reading adventure time! For improving reading skills in children with visual impairments', *Journal of Visual Impairment & Blindness*, vol. 114, no. 2, pp. 88–100. https://doi.org/10.1177/0145482X20913128.
Kortesluoma, RL, Punamäki, RL & Nikkonen, M 2009, 'Hospitalised children drawing their pain: The contents and cognitive and emotional characteristics of pain drawings', *Journal of Child Health Care*, vol. 12, no. 4. https://doi.org/10.1177%2F1367493508096204.
Lascaratou, C 2007, *The Language of Pain*, Jon Benjamins Publishing Company: Philadelphia, PA.
McCormicK, E 2012, *Change for the Better*, SAGE: London.
Medway NHS Foundation Trust 2020/21, *Quality report 2020–2021*. www.medway.nhs.uk/about-us/publications/Performance%20Clinical%20Research%20CTP/2020-21%20-%20Quality%20Account%20-%20FINAL.pdf.
Pelander, T & Leino-Kilpi, H 2010, 'Children's best and worst experiences during hospitalisation', *Scandinavian Journal of Caring Sciences*, vol. 24, no. 4. https://doi.org/10.1111/j.1471-6712.2010.00770.x.
Scarry, E 1985, *The Body in Pain: The Making and Unmaking of the World*, Oxford University Press: Oxford.
Sextou, P 2016, *Theatre for Children in Hospital: The Gift of Compassion*, Intellect: Bristol.
Sextou, P & Hall, S 2015, 'Hospital theatre promoting child wellbeing in cardiac and cancer units', *Applied Theatre Research*, vol. 3, no. 1, pp. 67–84.
Sextou, P & Hall, S 2015, 'Theatre & community: Bedside theatre promoting child wellbeing in cardiac and cancer units', *Applied Theatre Research*, vol. 3, no. 1. www.academia.edu/8667175/
Thompson, J 2005, *Digging up Stories. Applied Theatre, Performance, and War*, Manchester University Press: Manchester.
Wheatley, VJ & Baker, JI 2007, 'Please, I want to go home: Ethical issues raised when considering the choice of place of care in palliative care, *Postgraduate Medical Journal*, vol. 83. https://pmj.bmj.com/content/83/984/643.citation-tools.
Wilson, M 2022, *Storytelling-Arts for Health*, Blackwell's: London.
Winston's Wish 2020, *Charter for bereaved children*. https://winstonswish.myshopify.com/products/the-charter-for-bereaved-children.
Yang, Y, Zhang, M, Sun, Y, Peng, Z, Zheng, X & Zheng, J 2022, 'Effects of advance exposure to an animated surgery-related picture book on preoperative anxiety and anaesthesia induction in preschool children: A randomised control trial', *BMC Paediatrics*, vol. 22, no. 92. https://doi.org/10.1186/s12887-022-03136-1.

4
APPLIED PERFORMANCE, PUPPETRY AND HOSPITAL TUITION

This chapter will explore the benefits of applied theatre to children's tuition in paediatrics and their engagement with learning through puppets. It will draw on 'Bird Island', an example of my applied theatre practice in child healthcare evaluated from the hospital teachers' perspective and my reflections. This part of the book draws on my previous publication in a peer-reviewed journal that has been reworked for the needs of this book with permission (2022). However, the language I use to describe the methods and findings of this study does not always conform to an expected technical language, so I keep it in the same writing style as the book. Without this article, the reader would have less access to research evidence on the impact of applied theatre in paediatrics on children's ability to relax, communicate their needs, share emotions and engage with learning during illness. I will ask if applied theatre practice could bring a solution to this problem. The focus of the chapter is not on performance as a primary tool for schoolwork but instead as an artistic product with inherent opportunities for expansion in education that the teachers could benefit from. Therefore, I will investigate the engagement with hospital tuition as a 'by-product' of applied theatre in paediatrics. The chapter will conclude with my reflections on the use of puppets in participatory performance in paediatrics and its limitations and possibilities in clinical settings.

The 'Bird Island' project

'Bird Island' performances took place during school term days at Birmingham Children's Hospital and Heartlands Hospital (NHS) in England twice a week between 2016 and 2019. Performances toured on a rota between 10 am and 3 pm with a lunch break on various hospital wards, including Paediatrics, Cardiac,

DOI: 10.4324/9781003039341-4

Oncology, Haemoglobin Pathology, Dialysis, Neurosurgery, Paediatrics Intensive Care Unit (PICU) and Complex Care wards. The audience was comprised of children in-patients aged four to eight. The children suffer from various conditions such as infections, diseases, cancer, heart and kidney failure, and complicated clinical syndromes combining haematological problems with developmental delays and severe vision or hearing impairments. As in most hospitalisation cases, children who participated in the project suffered from physical pain, clinical anxiety and discomfort (Crane 2009). For many readers, the origins of the incidents during the 'Bird Island' project may be close to their experiences, and they may feel vulnerable. For this reason, I will use the teachers' words who describe what they saw in the hospital wards from their professional and, thus, neutralised perspective. I will focus on the facts as a subject in their own right. In other words, although the illness is inevitably centre stage, my research explores and investigates the nature of story making, creativity, imagination and the relationships between the child and the story characters even when impaired by illness. The point is to bring potentially overwhelming research evidence about sick children to the readers in ways that do not affect someone that knew and loved children with illness. However, illness and pain may overpower parts of the discussion of my findings, yet with respect.

Lollie the rough collie and the magic kiss

'Lollie the rough collie and the magic kiss' is a real story about Sax, our blond family collie dog, that happened to me when I was little. Sax came as a puppy to me in a cardboard box and changed my life forever. In the story, Puppet Sam stays in the hospital. When Sam feels lonely or sad, she dreams of adventures with an imaginary dog who hears the name Lollie (Sextou 2018). Sam and Lollie watch the sunset together; they make castles in the sand, run after seagulls and share the most delicious ice cream. However, in one of Sam's dreams, Lollie gets stung by bees. The dog cries, and her tears become pearls. The sky turns grey, the leaves fall from the trees and the girl feels anxious. The following day, Sam tells her mother about her dream. The mother reassures her that dogs recover well after a few days of medical treatment and care. She also mentions that dogs need love as people do. Sam absorbs this message, and the following night she dreams of Lollie again. Sam plays her part in helping Lollie recover. After internal dialogue with herself, Sam feels strong and brave to deal with this clinical incident. She takes Lollie to the vet, who looks after her. Sam holds her affectionately and tells her, 'it's OK to cry!'. She whispers in Lollie's ear, 'All I can do is love you', and gives her a warm, adoring kiss. As in all stories, magic works. The kiss is transformative and brings Lollie back to her old self. In no time, Lollie jumps around barking and licking Sam's face. The sun comes out, and the trees blossom. The following day, Sam finds a pearl tattoo on her skin to remind her of Lollie and the outstanding achievements of love (Appendix B: The story).

Feeling worried in paediatrics

Lerwick (2016) argues that hospitalisation is an anxiety-provoking experience affecting a child's emotional development. Children are confused in unknown medical environments. Because caregivers are taking over control of their bodies, they feel a loss of autonomy and control. In Lerwick's research, coping behaviours differ from child to child; therefore, children may need additional assistance in regaining a sense of control. Lerwick suggests that choices foster personal power in children and can encourage a strong internal locus of control during their treatment. Pain catastrophising in young children is closely related to stress in the surgical context. Therefore, despite pharmacological advances, young children continue to find surgical procedures the most frightening aspect of attending hospital (Schechter et al. 1997), resulting in pre-operative anxiety. Untreated anxiety has significant implications for children's short- and long-term recovery (Fortier & Kain 2015), mental health problems with repeat anaesthesia, increased upset, nightmares, separation anxiety, eating disorders and enuresis (Rice et al. 2008). Helping children cope with pre-operative stress is highly challenging for parents/carers and even trained doctors/nurses. Thus, children may experience more significant benefits from innovative and creative explanatory techniques of non-pharmaceutical preparation and distraction from pain and anxiety before the operation through a digital arts intervention. Non-pharmacological methods such as observing children reading books at home ease operative anxiety in children (Agbayani 2020). However, using these methods in the pre-operative setting becomes difficult due to the limited time children can be observed, the hectic scenes of the Operation Rooms and holding areas, and the inability of young children to communicate their anxious state. Because of these challenges, there is a window of opportunity for applied theatre in paediatrics to increase the efficacy of non-pharmacological methods for clinical use in busy pre-operative settings, improve child and parental hospital experience and wellbeing.

Lollie's story addresses the phenomenon of worrying about illness. It explores the boundaries of understandable concern and its consequences on children under health-related situations. The tale of Lollie addresses the nature of bravery and friendship and the benefits of love and compassion to a child when anxious feelings attack a child in response to accidents, crises, emergencies and health/ill incidents. In the story, I portray my understanding of worrying as a response to dealing with an injury that happens to others. The story aims to create opportunities for the children to identify an internal locus of power and control that would help them regain confidence in roles in fiction. I used rehearsals to guide flexible performance while encouraging the actress to give the child ownership of the story and the freedom to divert from the storyline in case the dog's injury affected the child's emotions. With the actor's openness to experimentation, the performance was an exercise of human liberty. 'Hospital' exists in people's imagination as an environment of ill health, incapacity, vulnerability and fragility, as well as a place for cure and recovery. Theatre in paediatrics should, in my view, offer the audience flexibility and the opportunity to be connected to the clinical experiences involving distress as much or as little as they want and can tolerate. How performance is going to develop and end is rarely predictable.

The dramatic frame

O'Toole (1992, p. 26) describes entering a dramatic situation as 'entering a "play-frame" that provides some protection from external consequences for those who step inside it'. The 'imagined worlds' we create when we use bedside performance in hospitals are also 'spacetimes', to use Edmiston's words (2000), where children can use and explore moments and experiences normally unavailable to them. In drama, characters' lives differ from the real-life patient experience outside fiction. The dramatic frame allows actors to meet children on the metaphorical ground. It also helps the child distinguish between life in a hospital and life in a fantasyland (Sextou 2016, p. 31). In this study, dramatic framing creates multiple layers of sufficient emotional protection for the child. For example, the actor, who plays the storyteller's character, animates Puppet Sam as a 'mediator' between the child and the storyteller. As a mediator, the puppet enables empathic communication and offers emotional safety to children of fragile health (Astles 2020). In the performance, the storyteller performs a short ritual to help Puppet Sam fall asleep. She takes Sam in her arms and covers her with the shawl with slow and gentle movements. Then, she starts singing a bedtime lullaby and moves her body to the music. This ritual pattern is repeated three times in the story. Children sing alongside the actor to help Sam fall asleep. They know Sam is asleep when she starts snoring. The storyteller says, 'Sam is fast asleep now. She is dreaming. Would you like to see into her dream?' The child dives into Sam's dream. The storyteller performs an 'awakening' ritual at the end of each plan. She asks help from the child to count down from ten to one, and they together call Puppet Sam's name as many times as it takes to wake her up. This is usually a moment of many giggles and smiles in the performance. With a calming and reassuring approach, the storyteller immerses the child in Puppet Sam's dream. Dreams in our story aim to maximise the potential of fictional protection as the child steps inside them.

It might be helpful to explain what I mean by maximising the potential of fictional protection in a dream mode. Dreams are stories within the story that offer an extra layer of dramatic action and safety for the audience. In Puppet Sam's dreams, good and bad things happen, but when the puppet awakes, the dreams are gone, and the storyteller can discuss them with the child retrospectively with emotional distance. What happens in a dream is just a dream, so the dream parts of the story (the dog being ill) worked as protected zones from Sam's reality in the story (the dog feeling well). I use the old good storyteller's trick of embedding a story within a story. In Sam's dreams, the child can see that Sam's dog was bitten by bees and was in pain, but the difficulty is 'unreal'; thus, it cannot affect the child's circumstances as an audience. Dreams don't last for too long, which can be a blessing. Every time Sam wakes up from her dream, the artist assures the child that the dream in the story is over. Dialogues between Sam and her mother about her dog also take place for additional comfort and easement of any worries. Clear distinctions between dream–'reality' within fiction were made to help the child remain in the story's dramatic conditions as framed from the beginning of the performance. At the same time, children are invited to step in and out of dream episodes where illness is portrayed and presented to the audience indirectly. Showing illness through an invisible character (dog) is deliberate. Illness cannot be seen and described in the performance. Illness may vary from child to child. However, it is present. Within dreaming, Sam expresses her emotions to encourage hospitalised children to express their feelings. Dreams become deeper layers of fictional protection in drama, offering space for truths to be spoken and joy to be experienced.

Participatory puppetry in hospital

Puppets are used as an invitation for engagement and participation with the artist in Lollie's performance. There was permission for moments of interaction between the child, the artist and the puppet during the performance, with laughter and funny comments. During participation, puppets generated avenues of spontaneous communication and expression of feelings (Sextou et al. 2020). Puppets are examples of emotional protection in creative interventions (Adams 2008) that foster healing, engage the child, generate a detailed description of their experience and facilitate the imaginative creation of new meanings (Desmond et al. 2015). Puppets contribute to the emotional safety of participants who experience fragile situations (Astles 2020). I appreciate puppets as tools to engage children in the story, keep them focused and connected to fiction and use them as a source of playing and normalising their hospital experience. In my research, I found that puppets create a 'safe space' for both the artist and the child where they can communicate and express their emotions. Thanks to the capacity of the puppet to protect the participant when entering an unknown emotional place, puppets become tools of empathetic communication (Sextou 2016). Sam's character represents a sick child. Because children identified with her, the puppet somehow unlocked the children's hesitancy to communicate with adults and encouraged them to play with the story. It may also be that in the imaginary world of the story, children felt reassured by the puppet and opened up to the possibilities of the narrative. For example, Puppet Sam says to her dog, 'it is ok to cry!' Most children cry in hospital. Although this is an understandable reaction to pain, crying is not always accepted as good behaviour. In a sense, the puppet gave 'permission' to the children to be who they wanted to be without judgment. Although it was not in the direct aims of the project to offer children the emotional vocabulary to express and admit pain, some children did admit their pain to Puppet Sam. Potentially, puppets in performance could reveal children's dynamic information that could help healthcare professionals assess their pain better towards effective pain management.

On some occasions, puppets create a 'healing environment' with positive effects on child treatment (Cowell et al. 2011). However, we cannot and should not assume that all children who participated in the project had the same emotional experiences. Yet, the stories teachers told us provide evidence that bedside performance using puppetry in healthcare can distract children from their difficulties and help them move from their hospital reality to a less painful or traumatic one – a worry-free fictional world. In the companion of the puppets, communication boundaries can become elevated with care and compassion in healthcare settings. In my research (Sextou 2022), I found that the teachers expressed surprising appreciation towards instruments when observing the children's reactions. Actors reported:

> As soon as children start playing with Puppet Joe to find Lollie under the bed, that often helps the pupils to engage because play is normality for them, and they don't relate that to the hospital but watching the story, that it's engaging and they have the opportunity to talk and think nice thoughts it's a distraction, and that distraction helps a lot with their relaxation and well-being.
>
> Puppet Sam sang relaxing lullabies with that girl recovering from a heart operation. She had been reticent since then. I think Sam falls asleep three times in the story, and it was amazing watching her sing 'Twinkle Twinkle little star' again and again to help Sam fall asleep. She was relaxing without knowing it. The slow tempo of the lullaby relaxed her muscles and soothed her mind. She started smiling at Sam. It worked well for her, but even children who looked nervous at the beginning of the story, after singing, they started breathing normally.

In combination, the dramatic frame, storytelling and puppets serve as an empathic and caring media of connection with the audience. A gentle and respectful approach to children's sickness created a sense of care in illness that relaxed tensions and improved children's moods. Most importantly, puppets appear to be helpful to teachers as a guide for care in understanding what the children think, how they feel, what they need and what suits their needs. The use of dreams aimed to set up conditions of caring in fiction. Two teachers referred to the performance as a condition of care and protection. Teachers said:

> Children are shocked by what's going on in their lives. It's a challenge to get them to talk about how they feel. Sam's story is good fun. Kids love it and talk about it. This is good. It makes them more aware of feelings, I guess. The story created the conditions for sharing feelings through puppets. Puppets worked as their 'emotional shields,' a protective condition for addressing pain.
>
> The joy of the story was down to the fact that Lollie the dog was ill, but Sam is playing the child who was well. The story is like a tool for revealing illness, analysing it, within protection.

How teachers described how children responded to puppets introduces new information about the use of puppets in hospital tuition. Puppets were used as animated objects that provide a sense of emotional safety and make them valuable pedagogical tools. Fourie (2010) states that puppetry as an educational means enables a focused and creative learning experience as the children are playing in a non-threatening and non-judgmental way. Matt Smith (2020, p. 56) points out that 'puppets can enable us to have the confidence to be odd, as a puppet is always other'. It is ok for the puppet as 'other' to look odd or weird in a hospital context. I intentionally use the words 'odd' (borrowed by Smith) and 'weird' because I have heard children in oncology often use them to describe how they look following chemotherapy. Children related to puppets in the 'Bird Island' project because the performance employed the puppet as a creative agent and a mediator allowing children to connect with the artist through the puppet. Children accepted the possibility of staying creative and playful (like the puppet) during illness. Smith continues (2020, p. 57) that Puppet oddness is a great collaborator in unlocking imagination and 'creativity without conforming to types, models, or what is correct or appropriate'. The practice of involving puppets and objects in the 'Bird Island' performance approached children as creative participants and not as vulnerable people defined by illness. Puppets supported the transformation of sick children into co-creators and co-storytellers. This achieved a natural engagement with learning outside of traditional teaching methods. The 'Bird Island' project proves that participatory puppetry in performance helps children engage with learning and do more homework while in hospital. More specifically, participation with puppets in the 'Bird Island' performance motivated hospitalised children to engage in verbal communication and connect with the artist during the activity and with teachers.

Research

Children who undergo treatment may find themselves in a transition from home to hospital. Changes in a child's life to new situations can present challenges, such as difficulties in making sense of recent healthcare events (Jun-Tai & Barbour 2014). Thus, they often lose the sense of normality and their appetite for tuition. Children who miss school while in hospital struggle with learning upon returning to school and lose educational and social opportunities to progress (Ratnapalan et al. 2009). Teachers in paediatrics aim to help the child catch up on missed work, maintain their pupil-role, smooth the way for reintegration with their peers (Craigen 2014) and improve a child's holistic health and wellbeing (Desai & Pandya 2013). Teachers at Great Ormond Street Children's Hospital school argue that learning is still part of the hospitalised children's world. 'It's vital that they don't miss out on their legal right to an education while in the hospital and unable to attend school. We (hospital teachers) provide continuity and seek to minimise disruption so that academic progress and an interest in learning will continue, as far as medical circumstances permit' (Stokes 2017). I witnessed many incidents of children who resist connecting and communicating with teachers in hospitals because of their health condition and how it affects them. I am not saying that teachers cannot find their way with children, but they must work hard to engage children in academic pursuits.

Hospital teachers' views are widely neglected in evaluating arts-based projects for children in healthcare even though the arts are repeatedly enacted in paediatrics with their support. My research shows that hospital teachers contribute different perspectives on perceiving and understanding hospitalised children's worlds that can contribute to artistic ways of knowing. I thank all these teachers who have permitted their observations and opinions to be included in my article (Sextou 2022) so that their views can inspire actors in healthcare to look at their roles afresh. By understanding that hospital teachers contribute different perspectives on perceiving and understanding hospitalised children's worlds and needs, we can either complement or challenge artistic ways of knowing. The study involved hospital teachers in evaluating the applied performance of children in hospitals. I aimed to use the teacher's skills and voice in reading sick children's emotions, behaviour and responses to theatrical intercessions during hospitalisation. Hospital teachers witness stories of vivid imagination, creative thinking, bravery, courage and expression of emotions.

Steinke et al. (2016, p. 41) argue that the role of hospital teachers is especially significant as they 'attend medical and psychosocial meetings, engage in research more than traditional teachers, and assist in the coordination of care between hospital and school environments'. Further studies indicate that hospital teachers are expected to develop higher levels of emotional self-awareness, understanding of emotions and empathic feelings towards their students than mainstream school teachers (Hen 2020). Hospital teachers must be intuitive and familiar with their pupils' emotional worlds and educational abilities (Csinady 2015). I chose teachers as participants for evaluating the 'Bird Island' project because of their unique position on children's experience of play and learning, both naturally related to normality, their responsibility to evaluate activities effectively, and they know to do so. The aim was to explore the project's strengths and weaknesses from a different angle to the artistic view. I wanted to provoke innovative methodological pathways in evaluating arts-based activities and foster an inter-disciplinary dialogue between applied theatre research and education in paediatrics.

Semi-structured face-to-face interviews collected the data from a committed team of ten primary hospital teachers from the James Brindley Academies at Birmingham Children's Hospital. The study occurred in the middle of the third year of the project (2018–2019), collecting sufficient data based on the teachers' three-year rich pool of experiences of the project and observations. The participants accommodated the ward actors to meet the children's bedside in line with the hospital's safeguarding policies during that period. This experience of seeing these teachers watching the actor and child participating in theatre bedside followed by their reflections on the project with incredible educational insight inspired the current research. The study applies a purely data-driven qualitative research strategy using interviews. It is exploratory. The experiences of experts relevant to the research topic were explored.

I designed interview questions to investigate predetermined and unexpected topics. An interview schedule enabled studying the participant's view on the topic via a question guide (Howitt 2007). To elicit unstructured responses and generate discussion, a mixture of open-ended, scheduled (scripted) 'probe' questions relevant to the research question were used (McIntosh & Mors 2015). For example, from your experience of accommodating the 'Bird Island' project on the wards, have you noticed any immediate effects of the project on child mood/behaviour/communication? Have you followed up on the project in your teaching session with the child? How did the children respond to hospital tuition when you followed up on the project? However, I could not predict how the teachers connected with the performance, what stories they had observed, how they interpreted them and how they wanted to communicate them during the interviews. The data were analysed using the inductive thematic analysis technique to identify and report themes that run through the collected data. Words and phrases were grouped, which led to the emergence of themes. I also kept reflective journals throughout the data collection to ensure reflexivity in qualitative research inquiry (Ortlipp 2008). Thoughtful notes focused on children's participation, mood and behaviour in performance in response to performances. The study complies with the researcher's institution code of research ethics (approval March 2018). Hospital teachers as participants were approached via email and introduced to the study's aims, the voluntary nature of their participation and the estimated length of the interview. Participants were then invited to present any queries to the researcher. If participants showed interest in participating in the study, they were asked to express their claim to the Head Teacher of the school. Face-to-face interviews were arranged at convenient times for the individual, on the same day, at the school's premises. Interviews were recorded via a Dictaphone for transcription, and participants were informed of this before the researcher obtained their consent to participate.

Complementing artistic knowing

Interviews with hospital teachers in my research revealed five themes: communication, expression of emotions, engagement with learning, enjoyment and pain management, and calmness and relaxation. Social isolation correlates with emotional pain and clinical anxiety (Mintz et al. 2018). Pain is an unpleasant experience that the child does not always have the language to communicate. I want to point out that my attitude towards the problem of communication with children in hospitals is best expressed in Lascaratou's (2007) theory of pain language. She argues that we should not assume that pain does not exist when pain is not verbalised and that there is no suffering, physical and emotional when patients are silent. Although the complexity involved in the experience of pain is not the topic of this chapter, it is necessary to acknowledge that pain, as a dominant element of the hospital experience, exists both as a sensation and an emotional experience. Carter and Simons (2014) argue that children do not always have the vocabulary to communicate emotions to adults. Sometimes they are too scared to tell others how they feel.

Therefore, the best way to assuage their fears is by recognising and communicating with them. As Bolton observes (1984), the drama does not protect children from emotions but protects them from emotions, within the dramatic frame. Instead of telling them how to feel and behave, we included children in the story as much as appropriate for their age and level of understanding and let them be in the safety of the dramatic frame. Communication of emotions, both verbal and non-verbal, is a vital component of healthcare (Clarke 2019). Thus, improving communication with children through participatory theatre is an important finding that strengthens its role in enhancing children's hospital experience.

Teachers reported:

Children who have been quiet and withdrawn since coming to the ward come out of their shells" "Sam put the children at ease with the environment and allowed them to feel less inhibited by what was continuing with them.

Feelings of happiness and joy were common throughout the performance. Children talked about emotions they spotted in the story such as how it feels being ill.

Older children seemed to understand that crying is normal when they are ill and that we should all accept that. As Sam says in the story, 'it is OK to cry. It's great to have a story about emotions. It's educational.

These observations are essential to the study based on the hospital's awareness of the high-stress environment. I wonder, however, whether children had emotional reactions to illness. The original stimulus in the story was an illness that happens to 'others' (dog). The aim was to manage emotions and avoid 'triggered reactions' (Lazaroo & Ishak 2019) to illness. I wanted to create a distance to the suffering of the puppet within the safety of the dramatic net, helping children empathise with Sam rather than relating to the dog and, by achieving that, maintain control of the situation. Children were connected with the scene of the dog being ill. Because they experienced illness, they were curious to know whether the dog would heal; thus, in my view, they engaged in the story. The teachers mentioned that most children spoke fondly of Sam and gave her advice with solid words of encouragement to help the dog heal.

They seemed to understand the value of caring more and tried to give Sam advice on how to help her dog by saying 'give her a cuddle', 'take her to the vet's', 'give her a treat', etc.

A girl (aged 6) in oncology was shy at the beginning and didn't say much, but after a while, she took off her wig and smiled at Sam (Puppet), as well as at the actor, and then she gave her wig to her mum and felt relaxed with the actor and Sam being there. She even talked to Sam. When the actor asked her what they should do to help Lollie feel better, she said that Lollie was scared and wanted Sam to hug her, and it felt like she was asking Sam to hug her, so I prompted the actor to suggest if she would fancy a hug by Sam, and the girl said "yes". Children with cancer, you know, don't like strangers around them. That girl trusted Sam and found comfort in the puppet.

We should not assume that the girl needed a hug because she felt lonely, neglected or scared. I wonder, however, and want to explore what the spontaneous reaction to the puppet meant, what it served at that moment and how it helped that girl find comfort. We can stand that bedside performance can provide hospitalised children opportunities to express emotions.

At its best, the artist's use of theatre and puppets is an inclusive recreational activity and resource, a live stimulus. Could the teachers use the children's performance experience to build follow-up school activities and help children join in learning, especially those who don't communicate verbally or in different ways? Defining the terms 'knowledge' in a hospital context is difficult. Looking back at my years of teaching, I recall that learning describes the child's discoveries, achievements and understandings of the world through activities that children engage in. Children can learn alone or with others in school and other settings, which must be an enjoyable experience. Learning should also be enjoyable for children with long-term illnesses who are away from school for prolonged periods. Hospitalised children lose their social networks and miss their friends. As a result, it is not surprising that many children, especially long-term patients, are less able and willing to do the school work during their hospital stay. This is alarming because it leaves them isolated and behind in their learning. In interviews with the teachers (Sextou 2022), the performance influences their pupils' appetite to engage with them verbally in positive ways. On some occasions, the performance becomes a social event in paediatrics, which also helps with communicating, as in the incident that one of the teachers remembered from her time on the ward watching Lollie's story.

> *I remember a girl in the cardiac ward waiting for an operation. The nurse told us that she was anxious because her operation was scheduled for the afternoon of that day and that she spoke aggressively to her dad before we arrived. The project was just perfect for that child. It diverted her mind from her surgery to the story and gave her something to discuss. She also made her puppet and asked if she could take her with her to the theatre room. She got out of bed to help Sam 'travel' from her bed to the next child. She even made introductions! She was a great advocate of the show who wanted every child in the room to meet Sam and play with Lollie. When the actor passed her bed to walk out of the ward, the girl looked at her mom and said, 'mommy can we bake cookies for Lollie?' She used her colourful cookware play set to cook for Lollie with help from her mom and then agreed to take Lollie on a train journey to breathe fresh air and have a picnic in the countryside.*

Some children first engaged with the artist, and then recalled the performance experience with the teacher and did some homework.

> *We have seen some children have shown more communication skills when the puppet and tree have been around and more appetite for sitting with the teacher and doing homework.*

> *I know they relate the performance to happy personal experiences and travel outside the hospital, which relaxes them. So as an observer, then I can go, oh, you've just talked about that, I can tick that off that one, you are engaging with an unfamiliar adult; two, you are engaging with a story, three, you are using your imagination, but you are also relating to personal experience, which is knowledge of the wider world.*
>
> *It's been interesting, helpful to our teaching, and we have used lots of text to discuss and try getting some communication through charts and things with children during their hospitalisation.*

A boy aged five and his family found inspiration in the performance that led to the child's engagement with storytelling afterwards.

> *Lollie's story was inspirational for my pupil (age 5) and his family. They were thoroughly engaged with the actress and puppet throughout the sessions. In fact, not only did he love the story, but he loved the puppet's hair and pulled the puppet's face toward him while the story was being told. Both pupil and parent loved the story session and the relaxing atmosphere the prop created on the ward. It was the sun to hear my pupil retelling the story from memory. The whole intervention engaged him in literacy without even knowing it.*

The teachers telling their experience demonstrates enthusiasm and the benefits of participatory theatre as an educational tool in paediatrics.

The perception and management of pain in paediatrics are complicated by how pain is identified and communicated from child to parents and from parents to nurses or teachers (Carter & Simons 2014). In teachers' views, the 'Bird Island' project offered the children opportunities for a 'happy escape' from the hospital, replacing boredom with action and helping with pain management through imagination.

> *Jonathan imagined vibrant, happy images of Sam playing on the beach with her dog on a sunny day. Children have a healthy imagination and enjoy stories because they apply their imagination to visualise other worlds and escape in places where they feel safe and relaxed.*
>
> *It was quite a moving experience for the staff on the ward to watch a child who was very poorly engaged in a session. After an initial refusal, the child saw the tree and was captivated by it. After some discussion with me about what he could see, he agreed to listen to the performance and became immersed in it very quickly. For twenty minutes, the actor was able to discuss things that the child liked; they talked about their own experiences, his favourite toy, and seaside visits. This performance acted as a form of escapism for this child. The nursing staff commented on how beautiful it was when they began to sing and talk, as this was the first time the child had spoken to anybody that day. On that day, we saw a glimmer of the child we all knew.*

Hospital teachers experience the nervousness of teaching a child bedside with no energy, desire or willingness to do homework when they feel pain. In the example described earlier, the teacher reflects on the story as a pain management tool for making 'escapism' from pain possible. However, Lollie's story is not an obvious pain story. It is not written to portray or represent pain in fiction. The word pain is used only once in the story. The story is about love and compassion and how these qualities can affect people's relationships when facing difficulties such as illness. But, because the pupils are residents of a clinical setting, the teacher focuses on the child's suffering.

Interestingly, the etymology of pain contradicts every contemporary medical definition. Yet it is not surprising that the teachers use 'happy' and 'happiness', in what may seem to be overstatements, as they strive to talk about children in pain. In a way, such overstatements prove how attentive the teachers are to the children's emotional experiences. Nevertheless, it is hard to conclude that teachers understand how children experience pain and how they benefit from their performance in solving pain management issues. But they appreciate the relaxation benefits of performance for the children, giving them a focus other than their health condition through breathing. In the teacher's words,

> Because children are not used to being here so for them, the story, a friendly face, coming along with a puppet, and the tree, it's all very non-medical, it's not frightening – which is kind of what we as teachers are, it's relaxing.

Peterson and Shigetomi (2006) argue that relaxation helps children prepare for medical or surgical procedures as a coping technique that minimises clinical stress and anxiety. In the accounts discussed here, gentle and casual interactions with artists through puppets or puppets animated by artists can help children relax. The claim here is that relaxation may be achieved by the soothing voice of the storyteller or the friendliness of the puppet, or a combination of both.

I witnessed moments of joy and relaxation with children and moments of ambiguity in performance when children were not responding and remained silent. These stories of Emma, Katarina and Azeeb reveal what I witnessed in complex and critical paediatric care units during the 'Bird Island' project. I share them hoping that the stories will illustrate the value of synergy in approaches to being present with the child and the parent/carer in most difficult situations. All names have been removed and replaced with fictional ones, and children's ages have been faked to appreciate confidentiality.

Emma's story

We met Emma, an eight-year-old patient, and her mother, resting quietly on the ward. Emma was a child suffering from 'locked-in' syndrome. In medical dictionaries, the syndrome is also known as coma vigilante, a state of unconsciousness from which one cannot be aroused. However, the mind of the patient is fully functioning. The syndrome is a rare neurological condition typically caused by a lesion in the pons, effectively the part of the brain stem that acts as a bridge between the brain and body. In its 'classical form', those children lose control of all bodily functions and can only move their eyes up and down or blink to open up lines of communication with others (Chisholm & Gillett 2005). They cannot move, but they are fully conscious. In Emma's case, the child pushed the lower part of one arm; she smiled, blinked and rolled her eyes. During the bedside performance, Emma was staring at the Puppet Sam. Her eyes followed the tool around the room. From watching Emma's reactions during the show, it was evident that the child connected with the puppet and was stimulated to communicate with her environment. For the needs of the performance, the actor brought a portable tree with prop bees, birds and butterflies next to the child's bed and plugged it in. The fairy lights on the tree also got her attention, and she blinked when asked if she liked them. The storyteller spent extra time with Emma after the performance. She covered Emma with the sensory blanket, which had stitched butterflies and bees made of various fabrics-surfaces. Emma touched the soft felt-made bees. She blinked to respond to the stimulus. Mum said that this was an indication of happiness. The storyteller sang the lullaby to Emma once more, and Emma looked up to the right again. Mum was pleased to see her child responding and communicating with her where the words were unavailable. I was present, and I felt rewarded by Emma's enjoyment and her mother's feedback. I discussed Emma's experience with her allocated hospital teacher. We acknowledged that we would never know exactly what Emma was thinking during the story. Still, we know that she enjoyed it, stimulating her to communicate with her surroundings. How Emma interacted with Puppet Sam raises a significant prospect: how can one use intimate theatrical performance to help a child, who is generally unable to communicate with the outside world, respond to the environment and experience enjoyment? Mum reported, 'Emma enjoyed the show. She was fully focused on the performance and smiled during the musical parts'. The mother also explained that Emma looks upright when she wants to communicate happiness and satisfaction. She did that repetitively during the performance. According to her mother, Emma was fully aware of what was happening around her, but she needed a 'nudge' (a strong stimulus) to express her thoughts and emotions in her way. From watching Emma's reactions during the show, it was evident that the child connected with the puppet and was stimulated to communicate with her environment.

Katarina's story

We visited Katarina in PICU many times throughout the year. She was reluctant to engage in conversation. One of the difficulties in communication with that girl was that she did not speak much English. So we sang her a song and interacted on her terms. Over time, she could sing with the puppet and giggle at the story. She would recognise colours from the tree and make paintings of butterflies from the tree and various story scenes. Katarina listened to the story one day but remained quiet while lying in bed. She would only speak with a whisper when invited to engage. We later learned midway through the performance that she would soon be taken to the theatre. From the teacher's point of view, the project's benefits were doubled for a child in anticipation of surgery. 'The show engaged her with fun activities and distracted her from her situation'. Katarina started coming out of her shell when engaging with Lollie, the imaginary dog, throwing the ball for her and giving her cuddles and a big kiss. She smiled at the puppet and played as usual while the actress tried to keep her relaxed. On another day, Katarina would hide under her blanket whenever anyone apart from her parents came to see her, only peeking out occasionally to see what was going on or to reach for her toys. When a nurse came and disconnected her from the machine, she darted off to run up and down the ward after being cooped up in bed for so long. At that time, she spotted the puppet and tree entering the community. The girl returned to bed enthusiastically and listened to the story with the other patient and her mum. She participated in joy and laughter and had many suggestions for Lollie to calm her dog. Afterwards, she made objects and characters out of clay. Her teacher commented that that was the longest time she had interacted with anyone in one session.

Azeeb's story

We met Azeeb at the hospital, awaiting a transplant. His teacher informed me that the boy also had learning difficulties limiting his world understanding. We observed low concentration, lack of ability to recognise and name objects; limited verbal communication and interaction with adults; difficulty making connections between words and pictures. We performed 'Lollie' to him seven times within the school year: At the beginning, the child did not recognise any of the birds, bees, butterflies and cherries on the portable tree that we used in our performance. He could not imagine a dog that was not physically present. He was, however, looking at the tree, a portable artistic installation, for a few seconds and then moved their attention down to the floor and back to the tree for a while. This happened many times. To make a positive difference in this child's experience, the hospital teacher and teacher assistant decided to support him in making connections between the characters. The storyteller gave the child a pack with a brand-new dog hand puppet and encouraged him to use it to imagine the dog during the performance. The child kept the dog after the show and practised it with our assistance. We performed to Azeeb again a month later. I observed that he used his dog puppet to interact physically with Puppet Sam and started making a connection with her. This was evident by watching him smiling at Puppet Sam and reaching out to touch her hair. He clapped his hands when the puppet was singing and pointed at the tree when Sam asked questions about bees and butterflies. After a few months, I observed more improvements. For example, Azeeb could recognise the birds and the bees on the tree, and he would sing the lullaby with Puppet Sam. He would make the sound 'bzzzzzzz' for the bees and even dance on the bed excitedly. That child who did not speak and recognise anything from the story could now give simple commands to the dog 'sit', 'stay', 'up', 'down'. He laughed, cheered up and enjoyed the performers' time in hospital. According to his hospital teacher, the child had made progress in concentration, recognition, communication and interaction by the end of the school year. Although the project cannot possibly claim the credits for all the progress, it helped the child be 'happier' (and I use the word because the teachers used it). The hospital teacher also reported following up on Lollie's story with Azeeb. He became more willing to work with them on the story bedside and more confident in modelling clay. The child's mother said she was impressed by the child's improvement over time. However, it is not known what the lasting benefits of the performance are on the child after the end of the project.

How each child relaxes is very personal because the experience of stress involves one's thoughts and emotions. A child in the hospital may think that they can't adequately handle the clinical stressors they are facing, such as thoughts about separation from family and friends, isolation, medical tests in anticipation of surgery, physical pain and so on, and experience feelings of fear, sometimes intense and irrational (Jun-Tai & Barbour 2014). These can accompany and even perpetuate children's stress response to the hospital environment. Because not all children have strategies to cope with clinical stress, it is essential to learn how to manage it healthily. An experienced artist can assist hospitalised children in relaxing through multiple creative ways such as play and interaction with puppets. 'Multiple' refers to numerous artistic tools and stimuli such as puppets. However, when extreme fears and anxieties are revealed through playing with puppets, qualified therapists can then give appropriate responses.

I give no guidelines, but I assert that there is 'therapeutic' potential in puppets within applied theatre practice, as I discussed in Chapter 1, which places the responsibility on the artist to normalise children's hospital experience through acting without crossing over into the therapy profession. Puppet Sam and Lollie's story comes with no intention of therapy. But because both the story and the audience share experiences of illness, and because the puppet creates opportunities for expressing feelings, it is necessary to appreciate the caring qualities of the actor. Actors are not qualified to treat children's emotional needs and restore their potential traumatic experiences through performance. I am not arguing for using stories that children cannot relate to or not using puppets in paediatrics, but only that we should construct puppetry in paediatrics from a precise awareness of the potential therapeutic possibilities it creates.

References

Adams, S 2008, 'Banishing Goods and Taits: The story of narrative therapy use in a grade three classroom', *Relational Child & Youth Care Practice*, vol. 21, no. 1, pp. 42–46.

Agbayani, C-JG 2020, 'Non-pharmacological methods of reducing perioperative anxiety in children', *BJA Education*, vol. 20, no. 12. https://pubmed.ncbi.nlm.nih.gov/33456927/.

Astles, C 2020, 'Walk in/walk as my shoes: Puppetry and prosocial empathy in healthcare', *Journal of Applied Arts & Health*, vol. 11, no. 1–2, pp. 29–47.

Bolton, G 1984, *Drama as Education: An Argument for Placing Drama at the Centre of the Curriculum*, Longman: London.

Carter, B & Simons, J 2014, *Stories of Children's Pain: Linking Evidence to Practice*, SAGE: London.

Chisholm, N & Gillett, G 2005, 'The patient's journey: Living with locked-in syndrome', *BMJ Clinical Research*, vol. 331, no. 7508. https://doi/10.1136/bmj.331.7508.94.

Clarke, S 2019, 'Children's experiences of staying in hospital from the perspectives of children and children's nurses: A narrative review', *Nursing and Health Care*, vol. 4, no. 1. https://pureadmin.qub.ac.uk/ws/portalfiles/portal/200399954/NarrativeREview.pdf.

Cowell, E, Herron, C & Hockenberry, M 2011, 'The impact of an arts program in a children's cancer and hematology center', *Arts & Health*, vol. 3, no. 2. www.tandfonline.com/doi/abs/10.1080/17533015.2011.561356.

Craigen, J 2014, 'A unique child: Hospital school – on the wards', *Nursery World*, vol. 3. www.magonlinelibrary.com/doi/abs/10.12968/nuwa.2014.10.3.1142625.

Crane, R 2009, *Mindfulness-based Cognitive Therapy*, Routledge: London.

Csinady, R 2015, 'Hospital pedagogy, a bridge between hospital and school', *Hungarian Educational Research Journal*, vol. 5, no. 2. https://dea.lib.unideb.hu/dea/bitstream/handle/2437/247637/Csinady_Rita.pdf.

Desai, PP & Pandya, SV 2013, 'Communicating with children in healthcare settings', *Indian Journal of Pediatrics*, vol. 80, no. 12. https://pubmed.ncbi.nlm.nih.gov/23378054/.

Desmond, K, Kindsvatter, A, Stahl, S & Smith, H 2015, 'Using creative techniques with children who have experienced trauma', *Journal of Creativity in Mental Health*, vol. 10, no. 4, pp. 439–455.

Edmiston, B 2000, 'Drama as ethical education', *Research in Drama Education*, vol. 5, no. 1, pp. 63–84.

Fortier, MA & Kain, ZN 2015, 'Treating perioperative anxiety and pain in children: A tailored and innovative approach', *Paediatric Anaesthesia*, vol. 25, no. 1, pp. 27–35.

Fourie, A 2010, *Puppetry as an Educational Tool: An Exploratory Study on the Perceptions of Foundation Phase Educators and Learners*, Thesis, M Tech Performing Arts Technology.

Hen, M 2020, 'Teaching emotional intelligence: An academic course for hospital teachers', *Continuity in Education*, vol. 1, no. 1, pp. 22–36.

Howitt, D 2007, *Introduction to Research Methods in Psychology*, Pearson Education: London.

Jun-Tai, N & Barbour, F 2014, 'Enhancing resilience in children and young people', in A. Tonkin (ed), *Play in Healthcare*, Routledge: London, pp. 93–110.

Lascaratou, C 2007, *The Language of Pain*, Jon Benjamins Publishing Company: Philadelphia, PA.

Lazaroo, N & Ishak, I 2019, 'The tyranny of emotional distance? Emotional work and emotional labour in applied theatre projects', *Applied Theatre Research*, vol. 7, pp. 67–77.

Lerwick, JL 2016, 'Minimizing pediatric healthcare-included anxiety and trauma', *World Journal of Clinical Paediatrics*, vol. 5, no. 2, pp. 143–150.

McIntosh, MJ & Mors, M 2015, 'Situating and constructing diversity in semi-structured interviews', *Global Qualitative Nurse Research*. https://journals.sagepub.com/doi/full/10.1177/2333393615597674.

Mintz, J, Palaiologou, I & Carroll, C 2018, A review of educational provision for children unable to attend school for medical reasons. *UCL Institute of Education*. www.hhe.nottingham.sch.uk/wp-content/uploads/2019/10/A-review-of-educational-provision-hospital-and-home-education-services-UCL-2018.pdf.

O'Toole, J 1992, *The Process of Drama: Negotiating Art and Meaning*, Routledge: London.

Ortlipp, M 2008, 'Keeping and using reflective journals in the qualitative research process', *The Qualitative Report*, vol. 13, no. 4, pp. 695–705.

Peterson, L & Shigetomi, C 2006, 'The use of coping techniques to minimize anxiety in hospitalized children', *Behaviour Therapy*, vol. 12, no. 1, pp. 1–14.

Ratnapalan, S, Rayar, M & Crawley, M 2009, 'Educational services for hospitalized children', *Paediatrics & Child Health*, vol. 14, no. 7, pp. 433–436.

Rice, M, GlAsper, A, Keeton, D, Spargo, P 2008, 'The effect of a pre-operative education programme on perioperative anxiety in children: An observational study', *Paediatric Anaesthesia*, vol. 18, no. 5, pp. 426–430.

Schechter, NL, Blankson, V, Pachter, LM, Sullivan, CM & Costa, L 1997, 'The ouchless place: No pain, children's gain', *Pediatrics*, vol. 99, no. 6, pp. 890–894.

Sextou, P 2016, *Theatre for Children in Hospital: The Gift of Compassion*, Intellect: Bristol.

Sextou, P 2018, *Lollie the Rough Collie and the Magic Kiss*, Tulleys Print Ltd (self-publication): Birmingham.

Sextou, P 2022, 'Theatre in paediatrics: Can participatory performance mitigate educational, emotional and social consequences of missing out school during hospitalisation?', *Research in Drama Education: The Journal of Applied Theatre and Performance*, vol. 1. www.tandfonline.com/doi/full/10.1080/13569783.2021.1940914.

Sextou, P, Karypidou, A & Kourtidou-Sextou, E 2020, 'Applied theatre, puppetry and emotional skills in healthcare: A cross-disciplinary pedagogical framework', *Applied Theatre Research*, vol. 8, no. 1, pp. 89–105.

Smith, M 2020, 'The sentient spoon as broken puppet: Celebrating otherness with performing objects', *Journal of Applied Arts & Health*, vol. 11, no. 1–2, pp. 49–57.

Stålberg, A, Sandberg, A & Söderbäck, M 2015, 'Younger children's (three to five years) perceptions of being in a health-care situation', *Early Child Development and Care*, vol. 186, no. 5. www.tandfonline.com/doi/abs/10.1080/03004430.2015.1064405.

Steinke, S, Elam, M, Irwin, MK, Sexton, K & and McGraw, A 2016, 'Pediatric hospital school programming: An examination of educational services for students who are hospitalized', *Physical Disabilities Education and Related Services*, vol. 35, no. 1. https://scholarworks.iu.edu/journals/index.php/pders/article/view/20896.

Stokes, R 2017, Teaching children in hospital: 'Learning is still very much part of their world. *The Guardian*. www.theguardian.com/teacher-network/2017/oct/20/teaching-children-in-hospital-learning-is-still-part-of-their-world.

5
CARING ENOUGH IS NEVER ENOUGH

Training actors on emotional skills

In this chapter, I endeavour to respectfully ask what it means to work as an actor in a professional environment dominated by illness? How does the actor feel when they are exposed to images of illness? I do not seek to criticise the artist's efficiency in surviving the challenges of bringing artistic interventions into clinical environments by asking these questions. I am asking these questions because I believe we can prevent emotional exhaustion by attending to the emotional needs of the artist who performs in the healthcare community. I will argue for the need to raise awareness of the value of observing and processing emotions in applied theatre in ethical and sensitive ways. The chapter draws on the importance of self-care for actors in healthcare and the emerging concerns about the effect emotionally draining experiences might have on the actor. Here, I will use reworked elements of these articles with permission to develop my thinking further. But first, I will present anecdotal poems written by actors as outcomes of reflective poetry on working with children within a clinical environment. The lyrics will be followed by a discussion about the importance of self-awareness, care and professional responsibility. Next, I will address the demand for training the artist to perform in clinical settings to the practitioner's benefit. I have written this chapter hoping that the actor's perspective becomes meaningful in the clinical setting.

Reflective poetry in paediatrics

The essential need I identify in the training of artists for health is culture change: change in conventional thinking about the actor as a 'vacuum of emotions' who hides their feelings behind a happy face to entertain people in pain. The argument is that we must train artists to be informed about the expectations implicit in the practice and develop both acting expertise and emotional resilience to connect carefully with paediatric children. This is registered as my empathic response to the

DOI: 10.4324/9781003039341-5

actor in healthcare being enabled to process and work through their feelings while performing with children in healthcare.

Performing in healthcare is a critical practice. However, telling stories in interaction with sick and injured children's bedsides can be a complex interface central to both the artist and the child's experience in the hospital. Working in paediatrics involves intense experiences, both rewarding and stressful. Preston (2013, p. 243) argues that community actors (she uses the term 'facilitator') provide 'emotional labour' in the form of care in their relationships with audiences during performances. Given the complexity of these environments, they can be emotionally taxing. Published evidence demonstrates that actors in the community worry that the arts-based activities might 'become traumatic or too close to their personal experiences' (Balfour et al. 2015, p. 117). The atmosphere in the wards can be emotional when the performance is interrupted by nurses and visitors, especially when they cannot re-establish the fictional conditions of imagined stories to continue the performance afterwards. Actors can be affected emotionally by clinical practice.

Poetry is an effective way to reflect on clinical practice. It explores nurses' perspectives on using poetry writing to reflect on critical nurse and medical practice issues when reflection can be challenging (Jack & Illingworth 2019). Jack and Illingworth continue that reflective poetry has relevance and transferability to a wide range of professional disciplines, where reflective practice is encouraged. I can see the relevance of thoughtful poetry to healthcare professions. Reflection is an ability that supports emotional resilience by enabling professionals to explore their thoughts and rationalise emotional experiences, which can reduce their impact on their wellbeing (Grant & Kinman 2014). Reflective practice in healthcare improves the quality of care (Koshy et al. 2017). I argue with my colleagues Karypidou and Kourtidou-Sextou (Sextou et al. 2020) that the artist will become better equipped to recognise their emotional boundaries in performance in clinical environments than those less attuned to their own emotions.

I worked closely with a poet to offer actors creative writing activities as a self-reflective learning tool about their preparation for performing in healthcare settings and in response to their experience of meeting children as audiences on the hospital wards. My aspiration of employing poetry for learning aimed to produce spontaneous conversations to reveal embodied applied theatre practice in healthcare wisdom. Hopkinson (2015) argues that poems may provide reflective insight into healthcare professions and stimulate and paradoxically encourage emotional distance, thereby allowing the dynamic nature of practice to be safely examined. Hopkinson explains how poetry may capture the complexity of nursing practice through its multi-layered nature, developing empathy and providing new insights. It incorporates conscious and unconscious experience to reveal a different way of knowing that is embodied and reflexive. With a focus on the power of expertise reflected through language, image and metaphor, actors worked collaboratively with a poet in informal open-ended group workshops where they had opportunities to scribble words, exchange them, co-compose sentences, get inspired by words written by others and respond spontaneously without an obligation to meet expectations and standards of poetic writing. The poet invited the participants to use the first words that came to mind while thinking of specific aspects of their role or the stories they performed. The creative writing activities took place during rehearsals, before and after theatrical interventions in the hospital for two weeks. These aimed not to teach artists poetry writing skills but rather to create a poetry-inspired relaxed environment for language expression about their experiences entertaining clinical worlds.

Authorship and ownership of collaborative creative writing are shared between five actresses who worked spontaneously together. The reflections I am sharing in this chapter are work made of many, not an individual product, except reflection 1, whose author prefers to remain anonymous. Reflections 2–5 are co-creations. There is not one author but scattered words on paper, expressions and relaxed reflections. There was no commitment to write descriptive accounts about their experience of rehearsing and performing in the hospital but to observe how they felt. Impulsive words were crafted in dialogue with their personal experience of practising and working in an environment of illness, their desire for making theatre with a social goal, the suspense of telling stories in acute medical settings and their fear in anticipation of dealing with images of pain and vulnerability. I am sharing extracts of writings to voice actors' perceptions of the hospital setting and raise awareness amongst practitioners about the actor's role in the hospital and the challenges and rewards of becoming an artist in healthcare. These writings contain reflections of the artists' state of mind put forth in a poetic mood, poetic manner even. The process they followed was engaging, inviting, seriously unstructured and open to possibilities. Still, these works are precious for their authenticity and insightful expression of feelings and moments of collective learning. I confess that I am constantly aware that the act of understanding actors' emotions in paediatrics is an ongoing and beyond my artistic remit process that encounters situations that are themselves complex and require knowledge of the human psyche.

Reflections

1

Blank eyes all around.
Beeps and clicks.
Silence.
And the smell of disinfectant.
What's wrong here?
What's wrong inside?
Does anybody know?
I can hear the seagulls outside.
I cannot see them.
But I know they are out there somewhere.
And when I close my eyes,

I go to that place.
The music takes me where everything feels alright again.
Where am I now?
Where am I going?
Always so many questions.
If only I knew then that the answers lay quietly inside,
deep in a place undisturbed by the pain and noise outside.
And the answers lay in the quiet voices of the people I would meet –
those voices you don't quite hear,
yet they speak to you somehow.
The hints and clues were underneath the words.
And the answers were always there.

2

I wonder in the ward
as I wander through the streets of an unfamiliar place.
To be home, to be safe
and warm and just me.
Anticipation glistens and tingles in the air,
like the first snowflakes
that fell from the heavens.
Where did they come from?
How long will they stay?
Can I capture one to keep just for me?
It fizzles and fades as it hits the ground
Submitting to the **brutal** *heat of the earth.*

3

I open the door, and the world is unknown.
Adapting myself to fit the space,
I find myself in.
Re-visiting the places I knew as a child,
I find them changed, altered, tinged,
as if someone has painted the colourful world
I knew with a soft, sepia brush.
I twist and turn and contract my limbs.
I distort my face to fit the mould,
to find the right face to show,
to please,
to entertain.
We are finding new ways to be me.
Learning new lines for my voice to speak,

for my heart to believe.
The excitement builds in the air
as the actors wait on the ward.
Driven to distraction as the people pile in,
one after another, a never-ending march of lost souls.
It is never personal,
purely medical.
I am straddling the line between one world and another.
Two so different,
never combined,
never meeting, until this moment.
As I walk through the open door,
I still feel I have forced my way in.
Show time!
I stop and breathe and whisper when I want to shout.

4

Connect.
I need to know more about myself more
to connect better?
It is being able to connect with the child.
The key to success.
Performance.
Finding connections
if you are open,
truthful and relatable.
It is difficult to be truly honest,
if you are uncomfortable with yourself
or do not feel connected to who you are.
Time.
Taking the time to let go,
be uninhibited by your fears.
Enjoyment.
Enjoying the process is translatable.
Knowing.
What is intuitive for you.
What you feel is right will allow you to be free and open to joy.
Laughter.
Happiness.
Emotions.
Exposed.
Emotions are powerful and new (?) and can be seen by all.

5

I look into the clear, crisp night sky.
Open, never-ending, vast space greets my eyes.
I'm filled with something bigger than myself.
The clock ticks endlessly on my bedroom wall.
Seated comfortably in a place readily visible for a rushed glance
as I run through the door,
again.
Distance does not keep us safe for long.
How far can we run from our fears before we end up back where we started,
again, having to face them?
I find no absolute comfort in distance yet am never at ease,
never able to breathe when I get too close.
I find my happy middle ground and stay there.
Safe, but inevitably stuck.

These writings are different from autobiography and fiction in that they are addressed to an unidentified person, possibly to someone that does not even exist. Their content is yet somehow personal, intimate and private, revealing mixed memories of anticipation, worries and joy as images are reflected from the floors of clinical wards. They add to my understanding of how emotional life influences creative works. The actresses' voices are valuable to me not just because I am acquainted with the artists who participated in reflective practice but also because they reveal how artists used words to describe their experiences. But, most importantly, they show that by allowing artists to express their feelings, we respect their need to attend to their verbalised emotional needs. Nevertheless, my intention in sharing those reflections was not to analyse their language or make interpretations of their emotions. Instead, it was to ask whether paying attention to actors' experience as performers in healthcare assists us in understanding better the nature of the artist's job in the hospital. They assisted me. Artists describe moments of anticipation before the performance, meeting with ill children, facing challenges, childhood memories, and experiences of pain, fear, joy and wisdom. It requires a lot of bravery to communicate the personal and subjective. The next question is whether actors have the emotional resources to process and 'digest' their feelings fully. Is it reasonable to care for the actor who interacts with ill children as much as one cares for sick children? The hope is that these questions provide a source of thought to establish a persistent need to explore the emotional experience of actors and audiences during the performance and develop helpful guidance for the actor in healthcare to support themselves and support children. In a sense, these questions can be answered only in the affirmative. As Femi Oyebode (2009, p. 75), a psychiatrist, poet and literary critic, says, 'Literary works, like all other products of the human psyche, are subject to the same laws: a writer's preoccupations are reflections of their inner life, which are in turn manifestations of their experience'. In my thoughts on how actors feel when they perform in hospitals, these reflections allow me to privilege language: learn to attend to the multiple possibilities of meaning and all the things about their emotions that actors kept unsaid but which were real and influenced their lives. I will use the shape of a labyrinth metaphor to explain my thoughts further.

Walking the labyrinth on the ward: a metaphor

Actors' entrance to perform in clinical environments often reminds me of a Knossos coin from the third century BC34 Banknote Museum at Corfu in Greece. The ancient coin portrays the mythical Cretan Labyrinth constructed by Daedalus to contain the Minotaur, the half-man, half-bull creature. A labyrinth is built in a way that offers people exits, whereas a maze is designed to lead people to dead ends. Thus, I use the labyrinth in my metaphor rather than a maze. And still, the labyrinth's concept represents a place of great danger where there is a potential risk, and the journey can be fatal without help. I am familiar with the labyrinth concept. The symbolic meaning of the labyrinth inspired me in the past to devise a theatre piece with drama students and design a theatre set as a symbolic space of mental illness. My colleague and I reflect on the student's project asking how the labyrinth was constructed of pebbles to portray the landscape in the characters' garden as a physical space and was treated as a symbolic representation of the characters' personal and emotional freedom (Patterson & Sextou 2017). In our work, we explain that through symbolism the actor aims to help the audience see the potential, to accept the dramatic convention, and by doing that, to get the possibility that one can mark the labyrinth with their footprints. As they walk in the labyrinth, they observe their inner experience, their distress and the appreciation of being alive through difficulty on a symbolic walk from 'outside' to deeper within their private selves. Characters in the devised play went through a secret passage. The labyrinth as a symbol fed the audience's imagination to be open to interpretation.

I borrow the labyrinth concept and bring it into the context of the artist's journey in clinical settings as a performer. Hospitals' architecture often mirrors labyrinths, but the hospital signposts can help patients and visitors find their way to the correct department and back out. In contrast, on a symbolic ground, the artist enters hospitals in anticipation of their meeting will sick children, as sensitively described in their reflections. However, there is no provision of 'signposts' to guide and help the artist walk in a challenging environment and walk it out emotionally and safely. Walking the labyrinth in a hospital setting may seem like a minor physical task. Still, in reality, it can be highly demanding. The artist walks the way to the child's bed to be present with a child who is in difficulty, possibly in pain and suffering, despite the compassionate care of nurses. The artist who performs in hospitals is faced with a personal challenge that will involve stripping away preconceptions and fears about clinical settings and treatments, acceptance of vulnerability, and developing intuition and wisdom in a deeper connection to life and illness as one aspect of life. The imagery parallels the labyrinth theme in the theatre, and the hospital is evident. Both include the possibilities of distractions, anxiety, fear or despair and a clear message that essential humility is vital to begin hearing and learning from those in pain. Finally, both suggest a positive transformative function and outcome of the experience as an expanded understanding of wellness and illness in the ongoing journey. Because performing in hospitals can enhance the struggle of the journey as it deals with the images of pain and vulnerability on the wards, it can become stressful. In these circumstances, listening to the artist's narratives needs to be a caring, empathic and compassionate process of making meaning of what can be complicated to grasp. 'Caring signposts' must be designed in some friendly-to-use form and provided to the community artist who is brave to perform for and with vulnerable audiences in demanding settings.

Caring for the artist: we can't pour from an empty cup!

I want to invite the reader to think about the artist in healthcare with kindness and ask how artists live with what they see and feel in hospitals, how they can adjust and what changes, if any, are needed to how they feel during performances. I would also like to add that I have worked with actors and puppeteers in hospitals who were creative and responsive, skilful and experienced. Still, they seemed to be carrying suffering and a sense of pain in how they looked at hospitalised children with sympathy or anger, especially those with life-threatening conditions, that I could not explain. Not everything has to be explained. But, as McCormick says (2012), it is not just what happens to us, but what we make of what happens to us, what we do with it and how we act. I feel that if the artist in healthcare wants to know their difficulties, they need to know them well and deal with them so that their theatrical practice is not affected by them wrongly, which is essential. To be excellent actors in healthcare, they must challenge the limitations (the Jungian 'shadows') that affect who they are and who they want to be.

In 2016–2019, I led a longitudinal research study with psychologists titled 'Training the Applied Theatre Practitioner in Healthcare: Exploring the Professional Skills', aiming to explore the actors' ability to deal with the challenges of the hospital location efficiently and professionally on hospital wards. Our research agreed with Moss and O'Neill (2009) and the APPG Creative Health Report (2017), arguing that investigations are necessary to train healthcare artists. In response to this demand, we were interested in how actors respond to witnessing emotional incidents and what skills and interpersonal competencies they use in paediatric settings. The aim is to meet the need for a better comprehension of the education needs of the actor in healthcare and contribute towards filling the persistent gap. I am elaborating elements of the study with permission from the publisher.

The study developed in two phases. In phase one, we interviewed actors in healthcare to explore the skills and competencies relevant to applied theatre practice in healthcare with a focus on training provision. Karypidou and I (Sextou &

Karypidou 2018) found that actors are required to develop an awareness of emotions during the performance, be adaptable to situations, be present in the now, stay calm, self-aware and emotionally aware, be professional, friendly and welcoming, and have empathy with the child, be sensitive caring, patient and reflective on emotions. In phase two, Karypidou, Kourtidou-Sextou and I (Sextou et al. 2020) gave open-questioned questionnaires to actors and puppeteers in healthcare to explore their training needs and opportunities in health and wellbeing contexts. The study revealed the distinctive demand of the hospital location on human emotions during theatrical interventions and the role of aesthetics in emotional protection. We acknowledge the importance of self-care for artists who work in healthcare because we have emerging concerns about the effect that emotionally draining experiences might have on the artist. We argue that the concept of emotional awareness and intelligence is fundamental to the artist when they work with vulnerable audiences such as hospitalised children and young people. In keeping with research about healthcare professionals' burnout and recommendations for dealing with emotional labour, we raised awareness about the need to attend to actors' emotions. In summary, we present evidence about the paediatric professionals' tense experiences caused by high levels of work-related stress and exhaustion when they work with children who suffer from chronic conditions (Pantaleoni et al. 2014; Mukherjee et al. 2009; Maytum Heiman & Garwick 2004), affecting their physical, emotional and social wellbeing (Portoghese et al. 2014). We are attracted by Koinis et al.'s (2015) recommendation that health workers could be trained to employ relaxation techniques and stress management strategies, get psychological support and attend counselling programmes. We also discuss the importance of emotional intelligence-related (EI-related) abilities such as resilience as a core requirement in paediatrics (Lee et al. 2015). Because artists may face emotional challenges like healthcare and medical professionals do, we are interested in investigating what personal, mental and emotional resources theatre facilitators need to feel emotionally safe in challenging settings (Hoggett et al. 2009). We encourage the reader to pay attention to the emotional labour and challenge amongst actors who work in caring environments and communities with high emotional demands (Preston 2013; Isenbarger & Zembylas 2006; Lazaroo & Ishak 2019). We conclude that artists need to consider how to understand their emotions rather than blocking them out as dangerous to their emotional 'safety'. I suggest that accepting the need to observe, receive and discuss feelings is needed versus the attitude of distancing from emotions when we feel uncomfortable with what we think. This would mean that the actor needs to observe emotions and their influences on their emotional state and how they experience and express these emotions during an intimate performance with vulnerable children. I wonder how an actor can control their feelings without disregarding them as an essential self-care strategy while maintaining their caring and compassionate practice? Future research needs to investigate the relationship between caring and emotional labour in arts-based work in healthcare. For example, the types of emotions artists experience when performing in hospitals and clinics, the kinds of communication and expression of emotions artists use in those environments and how artists manage emotions about social, educational and cultural differences.

Emotional awareness: an act of caring

One of the rewarding aspects of being an actor in healthcare is helping children improve their hospital experience, which can be satisfying. However, can we ensure the emotional protection and wellbeing of the actor are secured? Not all actors are likely to respond to the hospital environment because they have different experience levels. Some may develop anxiety about performing on sick children. Others may feel assertive during the performance. The claim here is that there is a need to consider the actors' emotional experiences, positive and less optimistic when they work in healthcare, and provide them with the proper care plans and strategies as 'caring signposts' to navigate themselves safely in healthcare settings.

We must remember that actors are exposed to emotional, caring and challenging situations during their hospital visits. One could argue that the dramatic framing is the actor's 'protective armour' against emotional engagement in hospitals as it uses theatre conventions of space and time. Theatrical conventions create emotional distancing and recreate the event's focus within the safety of the fictional world (O'Connor & Anderson 2015). Fictional framing is essential to all drama work with significant applications to hospital performance. It provides the audience and the actor with aesthetic distance and allows for reimagining worlds of illness into happier places. For the synergistic experience of an artistic performance to be effective in paediatrics, a connection of emotion is essential between the actor and the audience. It enriches the space of shared experience for the actor and participant.

In the study's first phase, actors reported the skills they need to connect emotionally with hospitalised children and distance themselves from emotions in performance, finding the right balance between fictionality and hospital reality, an act of in-betweenness.

> There has to be a degree of attachment, but you can't get too emotionally involved; you might get upset, I suppose you've got to keep that professionalism . . ., but at the same time, you've got to show your emotions as well so it's a delicate balance I guess between showing that side of emotion to do with the performance and that's acting as well, isn't it?
>
> In dealing with the challenging situation when a nurse rushes into the room, you must react in character, you know what I mean, not to break the aesthetics of the piece, just because something is happening and keep your distance . . . you need to be calm, considered with the role that you have taken on, need to be aware of who you are and who the child thinks that you are, not to break that fiction that you have created . . . .
>
> You can't get completely lost in your role and your lines. You've got to be concentrated on your role but also have a greater sense of awareness of yourself

and what goes on in your surroundings and know how to respond to your emotions . . . a lot of it is about Emotional Intelligence, understanding yourself, understanding the child, and how you might react to this situation thinking about how you come across to the child in that situation at that moment.

You need some quiet focus when lots of things are happening around you to provide the distance for yourself.

I wouldn't want to shut myself off because I don't think that's effective but provide some distance to protect me so that I can go on and perform.

In dealing with a challenging situation when a nurse rushes into the room, you must react in character, you know what I mean, not to break the aesthetics of the piece, just because something is happening and keep your distance.

I think you get yourself into a frame of mind before you go in. You can't ignore your emotions, you are in a role, so I think it is beneficial. You are not on your own; you can connect with the audience because you are in-role in the moment.

(Sextou & Karypidou 2018)

Actors' reflections coincide with Goleman's theory (2014) about focus and how it helps us handle emotions and thoughts and manage them for the better. In the context of performing to sick children, focus relates to the perspective actors can take that allows them to observe and monitor their feelings and remain professional during disruptive events. One of our findings was that focus and self-awareness are essential in developing empathy in performance with the patient's situation. Empathy differs from sympathy. It involves a deep understanding of the patients' situations. Empathising with the child in paediatrics may assist the artist who is performing in a caring and compassionate way and establishing positive interpersonal interaction with the audience. Actors' views strengthen the argument.

Theatre and empathy go hand in hand I think because you need to understand the people you perform to and so you can treat them like people opposed to sick children.

[. . .] just have to show to the child that you, as a person, understand they are going through a difficult time . . . and give them a chance for communication as an empathetic person and in a greater understanding a non-judgmental person.

if for example, a child is in hospital and we are performing, and somebody comes, and I must improvise, but I can see the child is distressed, I would be able to show empathy through my improvisation. . . . So, if you can show empathy in that moment of improvisation, and if you can improvise with the story in empathy, the child is relaxed, and they are like, the practitioners are right there with me, and we're in synch in a way.

These words have a particular resonance with the training opportunities that I am discussing in the context of this chapter. What focus, emotional awareness and empathy do is enable the actor's mind to deal with images of a hospital location and adopt ways of engaging with the audience within the conditions of fiction during what may be a stressful incident while remaining calm and professional. The above demonstrates that actors need mindful, caring and attentive strategies to deal with incidents during the performance. This finding coincides with the argument that being a caring professional seems to be an apparent competence.

The second phase of the study took a closer look at the training needs of artists in healthcare, including actors, puppeteers and therapists. We argue that our attention must be diverted from traditional training courses mainly about learning artistic skills to a cross-disciplinary pedagogical framework. The framework aims to enable artists to observe, reflect and process emotions before, during and after a performance with patients as theatre audience participants. The study design allowed the emergence of semantic findings that precisely portray the practitioners' needs as necessary for training artists for professional practice in healthcare. Responses by research participants highly rated the themes of empathy, emotional safety, emotional resilience, reflective openness and social awareness, self-awareness and self-reflection, active listening and the interpersonal skills of respectfulness, attentiveness, authenticity, humour, positivity, caring, enthusiasm, joy, curiosity, appreciation and love.

Empathy is the strongest category. Participants define empathy as a caring, compassionate approach involving understanding an audience's emotions and demonstrating that understanding. It also contains acceptance of the need of the audience to facilitate 'connection' with the performer through verbal and non-verbal communication. Therefore, we argue that artists must be trained to communicate effectively with their audience while maintaining emotional and personal boundaries. Achieving this balance is essential to protect the wellbeing of both artist and audience.

Emotional safety is another strong category in the data. Practitioners mention puppets as a tool for securing emotional safety for the artist and the audience in healthcare. For example, they see puppets in healthcare as excellent transitional objects, creators of a symbolic world between the artist and the child that help to create and maintain a safe distance between them and the audience. Therefore, our paper argues that training artists in puppetry could help them regulate the level of emotional investment, connection or distance in a healthcare setting participatory dramas.

Our study also reveals that emotional resilience is essential in applied theatre practice in healthcare because the location and the audience may require 'emotional strength', 'tolerance' and 'patience' from the artist to avoid 'emotional burnout'. The General Medical Council (GMC) expect doctors to 'demonstrate emotional resilience' as a core professional responsibility in their approach and defines emotional resilience as 'the ability to adapt and be resourceful, mindful and effective in complex, uncertain or stressful situations or crises' (GMC 2017, p. 8, 28). Throughout literature, emotional resilience has been defined in many ways, with the overarching category describing a protective ability to recover from life stressors without a long-term, negative impact (Grant & Kinman 2014). We argue that emotional protection needs to become a central aspect of the work of actors in healthcare, similar to the emotional protection training received by therapists. That is because synergistic performance in paediatrics is mainly based on emotional sharing, caring, warmth, compassion and understanding, all of which draw upon the emotional reserves of the artist. We recommend that training for the artist needs to encompass skills that will enhance their emotional understanding and resilience to ensure work-related wellbeing and job satisfaction in healthcare settings. In the study, practitioners also acknowledge reflective openness, self-awareness and social awareness as essential qualities in performing to vulnerable audiences. We argue for the need to train healthcare artists to employ reflective methods to improve self-care, engagement with the audience and their practice with clarity, insight and an awareness of their limits. I would argue that having emotional awareness and resilience as reflective abilities can benefit actors in healthcare practitioners. They can promote the ability to adapt positively to hospital-related stressors with images of pain and suffering. What next comes to mind is whether actors are equipped with adequate interpersonal skills to regulate their emotional experience in response to illness as health professionals are trained to do (Yilmaz 2017)? The study offers descriptions of the emotional involvement of the artist in healthcare in the practitioners' own words, revealing deep awareness of their needs and serious concerns about the lack of training for their profession.

Realisations to take forward

The applied theatre practitioner needs the capability to feel, explore and reflect on feelings (Preston 2013). Thus, accurately regulating emotions is a much-needed skill for a healthy theatrical practice in healthcare. We, artists and researchers in challenging community environments, can develop a healthy theatrical practice. By 'healthy theatrical practice', I mean an approach that is consciously open, calm, non-judgmental and compassionate for both the artist and the audience. When considering how artists connect with the audience and exchange emotions in synergistic performance, understanding caring and what it means for individual actors will help identify and respond to the artist's needs. Care is instrumental in relationships between individuals, communities and theatre practitioners. In Chapter 2, I presented the 'Rocket-Arts' project, where I argued for the need to focus on the child as a spectator in response to ethics, care and responsibility through the aesthetics in dialogue with participants to ensure the quality of the experience (Thompson 2015). Thompson and Fisher (2020, p. 219) argue that 'the arts can promote and perhaps produce inter-human relations with deeply embedded mutual care'. The concept of care does not contradict the notion of emotional resilience and acknowledgement of the actor's fear and personal adequacy in paediatrics. Suppose the actor is expected to be able to deal with emotional incidents in the hospital and remain on the role, professional, calm and relaxed despite the strong messages of discomfort that are experienced in the environment. In that case, the actor has a personal responsibility to protect themselves from the emotional burden as healthcare professionals learn to do.

For actors who work in acute medical environments, responsibility carries greater significance because they are exposed to dealing with their own emotions and children's emotions that emerge at the outcome of an incident. When they see children experiencing fear of needles or when they joy playing with puppets, for example. This leads us to think that actors may need to use their EI to find a sense of control and ownership of their emotions in overwhelming situations to develop a positive attitude towards the audience in performance while feeling secure within. Mayer and Salovey (1997) are concerned with the individual's ability to use emotional information to facilitate various cognitive processes such as information processing, the focus of attention and decision-making. They call this process EI. In fact, and this is by no means a statement to underestimate children's emotional needs in paediatrics, actors are probably less capable of facing stress than children, who are more resilient when facing pressure than adults (Goleman 2007). Perhaps, actors should develop a general awareness of emotions during the performance, including those of their own and their audiences.

In my view, our relationship with our inner selves, our perception of illness and wellness, and the best use of the opportunity to observe our practice and emotions are necessary to develop as professionals in healthcare and as individuals. How can the actor in paediatrics, for example, help children through the art form while learning to be cantered, collected, attentive, expressive, secure, compassionate and empathic? I find Goleman's theory (2014) about the importance of focus and awareness a suitable frame for those who want to think and feel about themselves and others. According to Goleman, focus helps us handle emotions, our inner world, and our thoughts and manage them for the better. In the context of performing for sick children, focus relates to the perspective actors can take that allows them to monitor their inner world and remain professional during challenging incidents. Lee et al. (2015) argue for the importance of the ability to read emotional predictors to the professionals' wellbeing and resilience. This means that efficiently adapting to emotionally demanding conditions could be a core requirement for the artist who performs in intensive care paediatrics.

These theories may be instrumental when we train artists to use their conscious minds to observe and reflect on their experiences in the community. 'We are all born with the potential for a healthy self which needs our observation, reflection, understanding and acceptance' (McCormik 2012, p. 11). Understanding what is happening inside the artist when working with an ill child within an intimate physical space is fundamental to building a healthy relationship with the child as an audience. We must remember that artists are not immune to stress. They may have experienced complicated feelings and fear about illness in their own lives. I have worked with actors in paediatrics who or their families had survived a severe illness and have had the experience of hospitalisation either directly or indirectly. These actors deliberately chose to perform in healthcare rather than in other community settings such as museums, schools or prisons for personal reasons. I recall an actress sharing her reasons with me: 'I want to give something back to the healthcare system for treating me so well and helping me recover from my illness in endless days in hospital when I was a child'. There may be other reasons for an artist to want to perform to audiences with the experience of illness, but this is not the book's focus. My point is that for some actors, the experience of illness and pain may be too close to their hearts. Therefore, it may trigger unexpressed or unprocessed complicated feelings when life pushes them into them. Performing in a hospital can be that push for some artists. Training the artist to understand their responses to incidents and images of illness in healthcare, developing awareness of self and others through understanding, as well as learning ways to cope can be essential steps in the further development of training opportunities for those who want to give something back to healthcare, and in other intimate confined community spaces, and that should be part of their training. These thoughts urge my desire to recommend further investigations in this field to understand better the training needs of actors in healthcare with artists as co-producers and participants that can voice their needs and affect the design of their professional training.

Who is the excellent actor in healthcare? A portrait

Earlier in this chapter, I defined healthy theatre practice in challenging community settings. Such an approach requires the actor to be adaptable to situations, present in the now, calm, self-aware, emotionally aware, professional, confident, friendly, empathic and sensitive to the whole experience, caring, patient and reflective. Anxious, confused, hypersensitive, self-absorbed, fixed-minded, inflexible, unconfident, stressed, depressed, dissatisfied and disapproving actors can prevent the audience from living the theatrical experience fully, ethically and emotionally safe. Suppose the reader is identified with any of the above and might struggle with the idea that it could be challenging for them to work in demanding community settings. In that case, they may find relief in understanding the nature of the job and the possibilities of change to challenge any assumptions or limitations. This chapter, then, might be an eye-opener for some.

An excellent actor in healthcare should have completed adequate training on artistic and emotional skills and reflect on their practice. He should approach audiences in clinical settings with kindness, empathy and compassion. Artists have their styles. Each artist has character, personality, strengths, talents, weaknesses and imperfections. What matters is their ability to connect with the audience, interact and build trust with the patient as a participant in the performance. Having read this book, the reader might already know more about the synergistic relationship, the 'magic' between the actor and the child in hospital, and be aware of how audience participation might be activated in paediatrics. Bedside, there are many openings for an intimate performance in confined spaces, and this is good because it allows actors to see their skills in practice. They can test their skills, observe them and experiment with voice, movement, gesture, facial expressions, pauses, pace, tone, colour, narrative and space. They begin to develop a repertoire of words and communications by doing that. No artist or practice is perfect. However, it is right to say that a good actor in paediatrics safely explores things with the participant within fiction and the dramatic frame, one that encourages the child to take imitative and ownership of the story they tell together without being patronising and overpowering.

I have come to a realisation from all the years I have worked with actors in paediatrics. The actor is not the bedside performance's protagonist but the conductor. Like the person who conducts an orchestra and must stress the musical pulse so that all the performers can follow the same metrical rhythm, in applied theatre, the actor keeps the performance moving at a steady pace, encouraging the child to keep moving with the actor at the same time. In a sense, and most importantly, the actor considers every aspect of the performance and how to make it as inspiring, engaging and relaxing as possible for the ill child. Then they work with the child bedside to make that vision come alive. 'Conducting' performance in a hospital is more challenging than playing one role in a performance in the theatre. A great actor must have theatrical instincts and intuition, but innate theatricality will get them only so far with children in hospital. Actors also need to be steered to align their actions with what the children are doing. The actor is the bridge between fiction and the reality of the hospital and the sense of what is happening in the performance (the bubble I discussed earlier in the book) within the clinical surroundings. The excellent actor in healthcare needs to be simultaneously confident but not overconfident, calm but not too relaxed, creative but not overpowering, entertaining but not overacting, and overreacting. Hospitals recast notions of actor/participant, healthy/unhealthy, leader/co-creator, active/passive, real/unreal and exposed/protected. In paediatrics, theatre with children requires a flexible approach that prevents fixed roles and secures inter-play and synergy of stories and emotions. In turn, the actor needs to embrace the insecurity that comes with uncertainty about the pace and outcome of the performance. This raises difficult questions about accepting stress and failure and self-criticism when acting in a hospital. Hospitals are healing places – it is a sad irony that actors who perform in hospitals may feel sick when they are confronted with stress. Why would an actor want to go through challenging experiences? I also often wonder myself.

The artist's professional self is like a seed in a pot whose growth depends on the soil ingredients and the conditions of the environment. Artists in healthcare cannot isolate themselves from who they are and their potential to *be*. Artists in healthcare, I believe, need to find ways to understand their gifts and challenges, as well as their reactions to experiences of illness and wellness, to survive the job. When artists face difficulties dealing with clinical incidents during the performance that affect their emotions, they have an opportunity to think, reflect and see their role in healthcare. These experiences allow artists to think of their training needs based on realisations in practice and learn from hands-on practical experience. Then, searching for suitable training for the artist in healthcare becomes a dialogue with oneself. This dialogue requires maturity, honesty, bravery, adaptability and expressiveness that evolve from constant interaction with audiences in the hospital and a massive capacity for adaptation. The actors are highly creative. They are the masters of improvisation! I have no ready answers to what professional training courses for artists in healthcare should be. But, understanding the difference in energy and flexibility between the artist student, with possibly restricted ways of exploring their deeper inner worlds, and the potential artist student that can reflect on their needs wanting to find a greater sense of meaning, to answer the question 'who am I?', should be at the heart of their training.

Artists in healthcare seek training for different reasons – to feel skilled and confident, to feel less anxious, to feel more in control of the experience of performing in clinical environments, to stop being affected emotionally by images of pain, to remain professional and support their wellbeing. Or perhaps they seek training because they feel vulnerable or exposed to vulnerability, unhappy during their hospital visits, or extremely happy; they see their role as powerful but are unsure how to handle it. Often, artists may not be entirely sure what training they need and what is missing and needs changing in established training courses. It may be easy to attend workshops and short classes on improvisation, clownery, puppetry, mindfulness, breathing and relaxation, and these courses can help. But unless the artist can observe their needs and look deeper into their experiences, 'ad hoc' training may be a short-term solution. We must recognise that artists are prone to emotional distress in acute clinical places and be prepared to look at our needs from a neutral and responsible perspective. Arguably, the degree to which we can moderate stress levels during a performance in clinical surroundings is subject to individual differences (Birks & Watt 2007). I would encourage the reader to look at the design of training for the artist in healthcare as a preparation for a journey: it requests an exploration of what artists need, think, feel and see to walk the path of knowledge.

References

All-Party Parliamentary Group (APPG) 2017, *Creative health: The arts for health and wellbeing: Report of inquiry on arts, health and wellbeing*. www.artshealthandwellbeing.org.uk/appg-inquiry/Publications/Creative_Health_Inquiry_Report_2017.pdf.

Balfour, M, Bundy, P, Burton, B, Dunn, J & Woodrow, N 2015, *Applied Theatre. Resettlement. Drama, Refugees and Resilience*, Bloomsbury: London.

Birks, YF & Watt, IS 2007, 'Emotional intelligence and patient-centred care', *Journal of the Royal Society of Medicine*, vol. 100, no. 8, pp. 368–374. doi: 10.1177/014107680710000813.

General Medical Council 2017, *Generic professional capabilities framework*. www.gmc-uk.org/education/standards-guidance-and-curricula/standards-and-outcomes/generic-professional-capabilities-framework.

Goleman, D 2007, *Social Intelligence*, Arrow Books: London.

Goleman, D 2014, *Focus: The Hidden Driver of Excellence*, Bloomsbury: London.

Grant, L & Kinman, G 2014, 'Emotional resilience in the helping professions and how it can be enhanced', *Health and Social Care Education*, vol. 3, no. 1, pp. 23–34.

Hoggett, P, Mayo, M & Miler, C 2009, *The Dilemmas of Development Work: Ethical Challenges in Regeneration*, Policy Press: Bristol.

Hopkinson, C 2015, 'Using poetry in a critically reflexive action research co-inquiry with nurses', *Action Research Journal*, vol. 13, no. 1, pp. 30–47. https://doi.org/10.1177/1476750314565943.

Isenbarger, L & Zembylas, M 2006, 'The emotional labour of caring in teaching', *Teaching and Teacher Education*, vol. 22, pp. 120–134. www.academia.edu/16642465/The_emotional_labour_of_caring_in_teaching.

Jack, K & Illingworth, S 2019, 'Developing reflective thinking through poetry writing: Views from students and educators', *International Journal of Nursing Education Scholarship*, vol. 16, no. 1. https://doi.org/10.1515/ijnes-2018-0064.

Koinis, A, Giannou, V, Drantaki, V, Angelaina, S, Stratou, E & Saridi, M 2015, 'The impact of healthcare workers' job environment on their mental-emotional health. Coping strategies: The case of a local general hospital', *Health Psychology Research*, vol. 3, no. 1. www.ncbi.nlm.nih.gov/pmc/articles/PMC4768542/.

Koshy, K, Limb, C, Gundogan, B, Whitehurst, K & Jafree, DJ 2017, 'Reflective practice in health care and how to reflect effectively', *International Journal of Surgery Oncology*, vol. 2, no. 6. https://pubmed.ncbi.nlm.nih.gov/29177215/.

Lazaroo, N & Ishak, I 2019, 'The tyranny of emotional distance? Emotional work and emotional labour in applied theatre projects', *Applied Theatre Research*, vol. 7, no. 1, pp. 67–77.

Lee, KJ, Forbes, ML, Lukasiewicz, GJ, Williams, T, Sheets, A, Fischer, K & Niedner, MF 2015, 'Promoting staff resilience in the pediatric intensive care unit', *American Journal of Critical Care*, vol. 24, no. 5, pp. 422–430.

Mayer, JD & Salovey, P 1997, 'What is emotional intelligence?', in P Salovey & DJ Sluyter (eds), *Emotional Development and Emotional Intelligence: Educational Implications* (pp. 3–34), Basic Books: New York.

Maytum, JC, Heiman, MB & Garwick, AW 2004, 'Compassion fatigue and burnout in nurses who work with children with chronic conditions and their families', *Journal of Pediatric Health Care*, vol. 18, no. 4, pp. 171–179.

McCormik, EW 2012, *Change for the Better. Self-Help through Practical Psychotherapy*, SAGE: London.

Moss, H & O'Neill, D 2009, *What training do artists need to work in healthcare settings? Medical Humanities*, 1, pp. 1–5.

Mukherjee, S, Beresford, B, Glaser, A & Sloper, P 2009, 'Burnout, psychiatric morbidity, and work-related sources of stress in paediatric oncology staff: A review of the literature', *Psycho-oncology*, vol. 18, no. 10, pp. 1019–1028.

O'Connor, P & Anderson, M 2015, *Applied Theatre Research: Radical Departures*, Bloomsbury: London.

Oyebode, F (ed.) 2009, *Mindreadings. Literature and psychiatry*, The Royal College of Psychiatrists: London.

Pantaleoni, JL, Augustine, EM, Sourkes, BM & Bachrach, LK 2014, 'Burnout in pediatric residents over a two-year period: A longitudinal study', *Academic Pediatrics*, vol. 14, no. 2, pp. 167–172.

Patterson, P & Sextou, P 2017, 'Trapped in the labyrinth': Exploring mental illness through devised theatrical performance, *Medical Humanities*, vol. 43, no. 2, pp. 86–91.

Portoghese, I, Galletta, M, Coppola RC, Finco, G & Campagna, M 2014, 'Burnout and workload among health care workers: The moderating role of job control', *Safe Health Work*, vol. 5, no. 3, pp. 152–157.

Preston, S 2013, 'Managed hearts? Emotional labour and the applied theatre facilitator in urban settings', *Research in Drama Education: The Journal of Applied Theatre and Performance*, vol. 18, no. 3, pp. 230–245.

Sextou, P & Karypidou, A 2018, 'What does the actor need to perform in healthcare? Emotional demands, skills and competencies', *Applied Theatre Research*, vol. 6, no. 2, pp. 107–119. https://doi.org/10.1386/atr.6.2.107_1.

Sextou, P, Karypidou, A & Kourtidou-Sextou, E 2020, 'Applied theatre, puppetry and emotional skills in healthcare: A cross-disciplinary pedagogical framework', *Applied Theatre Research*, vol. 8, no. 1, pp. 89–105. https://doi.org/10.1386/atr_00028_1.

Thompson, J 2015, 'Towards an aesthetics of care', *Research in Drama Education: The Journal of Applied Theatre and Performance*, vol. 20, no. 4, pp. 430–441.

Thompson, J & Fisher, A 2020, *Performing Care. New Perspectives on Socially Engaged Performance*, Manchester University Press: Manchester. www.manchesteropenhive.com/view/9781526146816/9781526146816.xml.

Yilmaz, EB 2017, 'Resilience as a strategy for struggling against challenges related to the nursing profession', *Chinese Nursing Research*, vol. 4, no. 1, pp. 9–13.

6
THE FUTURE
Questions and recommendations

This final chapter develops into three parts: a flashback of moments and arguments I shared in the book, the learning I gained from the COVID-19 pandemic and recommendations for change. Drawing on my practice and the 'From live-to-digital' developments (AEA 2016), I will raise some logical questions for arts organisations, healthcare providers and researchers about access to technology, power and knowledge and the production of applied theatre work in paediatrics. I hope this part of the book will implant curiosity and a desire to create a model where theatre and technology practitioners are free to pursue artistic work at the highest level outside of stereotypical work models and improve the lives of hospitalised children. I will conclude the chapter with a critical view; there is a need for change in the provision of the arts in healthcare and a need for action to ensure a sustainable future. Recommendations for actions by artists, healthcare providers, governments and local authorities are offered to argue for a more balanced healthcare system that will provide opportunities for the arts to play an instrumental part in healthcare during children's treatment and recovery. The arts are rich and powerful and deserve an equal place rather than playing the 'poor relative' role in healthcare.

A flashback: my practice in a nutshell

Applied theatre in paediatrics incubated slowly in my mind. It evolved through a lengthy process of leading, witnessing and reflecting on bedside performances in hospital wards. It has danced on the borderline between the arts and health, where the artistic and medical practices can ideally co-exist and complement each other while keeping their own identities, characteristics, roles and responsibilities separate. It has been both respectful and reflective. Some place on a 'stitched land' between reality and fiction, wellness and illness, personal and public. Sometimes it floats between expectations of the meaningful and extraordinary in stories, and

DOI: 10.4324/9781003039341-6

at other times, it remains within the zone of the expected. It tells stories and asks questions about the artistry of theatre in paediatrics, the language of pain, the use of metaphor in expressing emotions during arts-based interventions in hospital, the artist's power, the power of the child and the power of illness. It argues for cross-disciplinary partnerships between artists, healthcare professionals and hospital teachers, and raises awareness about the emotional labour and training of the artist in clinical settings. It never assumes or declares that adults have control over stories and performance, especially when working with vulnerable children in hospitals. Even though adults make rules and decisions for the child's health and wellbeing within their professions, it demonstrates that children have the right to the arts during their illness and treatment. It accepts that children's abilities can develop and flourish through practical engagement with the arts and processes of creative thought production, such as telling stories. However, it addresses that the right to joy becomes problematic during illness.

I define applied theatre in paediatrics as a synergistic, in-betweenness, empathic, playful, non-therapy intentioned phenomenon where feeling, listening and caring are essential qualities by which the actor connects with the child in drama gently and ethically. I argue that applied theatre involves diverse activities in creating opportunities for the audience to express their imagination and cannot happen unless the actor's imagination is unlocked. The intention is to appreciate the potential of performing and imagining in cooperation with children. This is where the idea of applied theatre enhances the experience of interconnectivity between actors and audiences. It moves into the realm of synergy, working collectively, sharing and experimenting with ideas. Theatre knows the importance of working with others to produce a unified effect. Participatory bedside performance at its best is a product of co-thinking in a process that is nurtured organically rather than being conveyed by the actor as an authority (Prior 2020). What is particular to the applied theatre in hospitals is its unique privacy and intimacy, which I describe as a fictional 'bubble', a private condition of protected space and time from outside interruptions and disturbances by hospital staff and visitors. Actors might want to sensibly consider how they engage audiences in the 'bubble' of their practice to respect participants and secure the stability of fiction within busy and noisy clinical environments. In most of my practice, the intimacy of the performance, flexibly constructed and gently performed, enables children to interact with the actor and play with creativity. In this way, the reality is not ignored in my practice; illness and hospital images are there; instead, they are normalised.

I believe that I have tried to warn the reader that some of the practices presented in the book might be mistakenly perceived as therapeutic practices. Despite the attention to the tensions between art and therapy, I argue that applied theatre in paediatrics offers opportunities for the child to express feelings, engage with learning, and gain a sense of joy and relaxation through the arts. I never argue, however, that applied theatre is intended to heal children's emotional wounds. In this book, narratives, puppetry, props, films, objects and toys become centre-stage participants in telling the story of stories in paediatrics inspired by theatrical magic and aimed at quality performance. I always search for a balance between using the art form to help children in need and making art that can move the souls of an audience no matter their health condition. I aim to combine theatre with other art forms and technology to outreach children during unprecedented times without compromising the quality of the aesthetics: the social purpose versus caring for the art. But, because theatre in a hospital is a site-specific performance, illness and healthcare rules and policies disturb the comfort of artistic choice. The audience is specific as the space, and they both demand responses to resolve the legitimate details of such an unfair battle between the role of the arts and medicine in healthcare. Therefore, while analysing applied theatre in contexts and illness settings, I respect the pain, the trauma and the clinical culture where the artist enters as an empathic and compassionate facilitator of artistic interventions-not as a therapist. Applied theatre practice restores children's agency as patients but cannot restore lives.

In Chapter 4, evidence shows that storytelling and puppets in combination serve as a caring medium of connection with the audience. Indeed, a talented, clever and engaging use of stories and objects in performance creates a sense of care in illness that relaxes tensions and improves children's moods. However, the intentional focus in using them in my practice is on the benefits of audience participation rather than mastery of handling overwhelming situations. It is also true that the stories in Chapter 3 could have been analysed more deeply by therapists who ideally would have worked with the children to whom the stories belonged. In applied theatre practice, however, we never dig up too deep to explain how feelings may be projected into puppets and objects and how toys may become vehicles for helping the hospitalised child to cope with their emotions and relationships with others. However, it is sensible to wonder whether to explore the possibility that metaphors that the children use in their stories may be relevant to their experiences – as discussed in Chapter 3. Given the experiences each child has had over periods of hospitalisation, we can understand that it is not impossible that applied theatre practice can bring children's emotions into the open within the safety of fiction. Research arguments and claims, assumptions and interpretations of the stories' meaning, purpose and usage in hospital settings have aimed for accuracy but may have been personal. Significance is relevant. What matters is curiosity and the bravery to investigate what it is like to balance on the margins of illness and wellness without fear within the safe conditions of drama.

In Chapter 3, some realisations about the role of parents and families in the arts in hospitals occurred in my reflection on children's stories. The work we offered to children extended the opportunity for parents to interact with their children and enhanced the parent and child's ability to employ the performance experience in other related activities. Parental feedback to my practice raised hopes for finding creative ways to integrate parents and families in designing and implementing arts-based projects as critical friends and advisors on the children's needs. Reflecting on the positive ways children and parents exercised agency is an excellent opportunity to explore what might be achieved by working with parents and children more systematically in hospitals. Without art departments and schools in many hospitals worldwide, involving families in applied theatre practice could be an effective strategy to support children and the arts in healthcare.

It is evident throughout the book that pursuing research on hospital wards has led me to appreciate the creative ways children use the clinical space during the performance, in contrast to their suffering. It made me think that the hospital experience cannot be precisely replaced or exchanged for anything because of poor health. The arts have no mission to cure illness but to offer opportunities for inclusivity and participation in enjoyment and relaxation during illness. Creative inspiration and artistic quality of practice depend on the artists, on whether they open their thinking about what illness is and open their hearts to those ill so that all children are welcome to participate in the arts, even the most vulnerable. If the artist senses the child's emotional needs and invites them to an intimate performance with respect and attendance to emotions, a synergy between the child and the artist will be created, and stories will evolve. At the core of the stories of this book are freedom of choice, openness to shared ownership and attendance. When the child connects, the suffering falls away, and the theatrical intervention offers excellent advantages – the joy of interaction and plays in a normalised clinical experience strengthens the children. Although applied theatre practice cannot fix or replace anything, it can allow the audience to be in illness with less anguish.

I try to show that applied theatre practice can make a hospital less daunting and scary for children. While it is perhaps less expected that children can still be playful, creative and imaginative during challenging situations, the stories of this book prove the opposite, which also proves that theatre made the hospital experience a little more bearable. Applied theatre practice can positively impact children's experience in medical-dominated environments when it is created with sensitivity and attention to children's needs and willing adaptability to meet them. Bedside performances seem simple, short and superficial, yet performing to ill children face-to-face and one-to-one is a demanding, complex art. It involves acting, improvisation and intuition. Rehearsed for specific populations and settings, bedside performances are imagined spaces for escapism, creativity and normality, and therein lie their benefits. Their best performances provide time and space for expression, play, interaction, communication, laughter, decision-making and learning. They support children's need to receive care through aesthetics in hospitals. We must acknowledge that the artists who worked on the projects of this book are brilliant humans.

In addition to being good fun for children, I aim my applied theatre practice to facilitate a sense of normality. The normalisation of the hospital experience happens because synergistic performances can create fictional environments in the child's imagination, distract them from the reality they experience in the clinical setting and encourage them to interact in playful theatre-based activities. Chapters 2, 3 and 4 describe these functions of my practice and illustrate them with examples of the 'Rocket-Arts' and the 'Bird Island' projects and how they have inspired children to tell stories. The experience of participating in stories about astronauts and animals travelling into space and playing with an invisible dog while chasing seagulls on the beach creates an illusion of being immersed in a fictional world and separate from hospital life. This illusion appears to have allowed space for expression and enjoyment through which children revealed their talents as storytellers. Although children are not professional storytellers, they somehow know what to put in their stories, how much emotion to release, when to stop it so it won't become overwhelming and where to end them. That is an act of a genius! Not all the children who participate in applied theatre have the ability, skill and capacity to make sense of what happens to their bodies, why they are in hospital, what treatment they take and how they experience hospitalisation. But most children know how to have fun. They play by instinct. Some of them travel in the fantasyland while also aware of their realities, being both in and out of it, balancing in-between the two worlds, possibly gaining the best of both. Children's stories are so precious as a tool for us to acknowledge their value and gain a sense of rightness by reading them. By 'rightness', I mean deep and truthful appreciation.

For actors to make a positive difference in children's health and wellbeing in hospitals, they must feel physically and psychologically secure. Chapter 5 explored what it means to work as an actor in a professional environment dominated by illness and how actors and puppeteers think when exposed to images of illness. Through actors' reflective poems and research findings based on my work with psychologists, I 'zoom into' the artist's efficiency to survive the challenges of bringing artistic interventions into clinical environments. Still, I have no intention of criticising them but to argue that by attending to the emotional labour of the artist in healthcare, we can prevent emotional exhaustion. Because actors can be affected emotionally, I argue for the need to raise awareness of the value of observing and processing emotions in applied theatre ethically and culturally sensitively. Part of the suggestion is to introduce the importance and necessity of preparing by teaching them skills of self-caring and empathy, compassion and caring for others with professional accountability. I argued that we must train artists responsibly, with sensibility and kindness, so that they are informed about the expectations implicit in the practice and develop both acting expertise and emotional resilience to connect carefully with paediatric children. I use the labyrinth as a metaphor to show that the artist who walks in the hospital is on a journey from outside the hospital (a sense of normality) into the labyrinth's centre (where the ill child lives). The excellent actor knows how to bring theatre (fiction) to the hospital (reality) and learn from those in pain. Together with the child and in dialogue, the actor responds to the child's needs with empathy in performance. We must remember how important it is for the artist to listen to their inner voices, what they need and how they feel, be caring, empathic and compassionate to themselves, and learn from refining their art with mindful attributes. This type of listening makes applied theatre practice a robust, effective, ethical environment and a safe space for interconnectivity and synergy with the audience.

Post-pandemic learning

The COVID-19 pandemic, I am convinced, does not mark the end of knowing about applied theatre, but rather it marks the beginnings of new combinations of professions, knowledge exchanges and experimentation, and it inevitably raises many questions about the future of applied theatre in healthcare and beyond.

The pandemic has not made it easier for artists to work with children in paediatrics. Since March 2020, when COVID-19 hit England, restrictions were enforced on visiting hospitals to protect patients and staff from the pandemic. The changes in creative industries, and society, were immense. The coronavirus pandemic has massively affected Creative Industries (Mak et al. 2021). The situation was a catastrophe for arts companies and freelance actors who could not find work without government intervention and support. As a result, arts-based projects were paused on all clinical sites in the country. Before the pandemic, hospitalised children had interacted with visitors, family, friends and actors-in-residence, helping them cope with the clinical stressors. However, during COVID-19, they often isolated themselves in the hospital. When vulnerable children needed the arts more than ever to support their wellbeing and normalise their hospitalised lives, they could not benefit from them for reasonable but still limiting reasons. Children in the hospital wards were excluded from opportunities to meet the actor bedside and interact with them through the arts as a creative distraction from illness, relaxation and communication with others. The restrictions of access to children urged my efforts to introduce alternative arts-based, mostly digitalised, interventions in hospitals to resist various limitations while attending to children's needs for enjoyment and relaxation. And still, I am aware of the chaos that the pandemic causes at all social levels, services and functions. It is beyond the healthcare systems' policies and capacity to allow non-medical and health professionals to visit patients under such severe and unprecedented circumstances. I would just have hoped, in an ideal world, that there could be ways to recognise the contribution of the arts to patients' lives when they needed it most during a crisis. I believe that having thousands of unemployed artists during the pandemic staying at home was a missed opportunity to support thousands of patients and their families in hospitals.

The complexity of the COVID-19 pandemic situation has triggered outbursts of emotional difficulties amongst children with neurodevelopmental or emotional problems and children with special needs. The pandemic has disrupted children's lives due to isolation from friends and exposure to increased family stress and violence, causing anxiety and depressive symptoms (Racine et al. 2020). The whole situation of staying in the hospital during COVID-19 has increased children's difficulty coping with pain and caused increased anxiety during hospitalisation. There are, of course, other factors than the pain that may influence the degree to which children experience difficulties in the hospital, such as lack of normality and homesickness. The copying process can be even more complicated when family and friends' support groups have collapsed. Singh et al. (2020) argue that enforced restrictions due to the pandemic, such as lockdowns and limited interaction with parents, carers and other support groups, increased their intolerance for uncertainty and affected their ability to follow instructions work independently and control their behaviour. Conlon et al. (2021) support this view and further argue that the pandemic and public health restrictions have hurt children's health and psychosocial wellbeing. This is the case, particularly for children with long-term physical health conditions, impacts those living with anxiety and depression, hyperactivity conditions or attention deficit hyper disorder, children with special educational needs and learning disabilities and children with chronic illnesses. These children may feel less confident about managing them effectively. They need additional support to adapt to routine changes and understand what is happening (The Children's Society 2021). The impact of isolation on children and young people's mental and emotional health is of grave concern (Meherali et al. 2021). The commitment to provide arts interventions to improve children's moods and distract them from loneliness and isolation in crisis is significant. It has increased the demand for new tools and methods of accessing and supporting vulnerable children's emotional needs, such as anxiety and depression during COVID-19. In many ways, the pandemic significantly influenced the methods and approaches to the arts to improve the health and wellbeing of hospitalised populations. It has created the time to think and the space to dream about the future of applied theatre in hospitals and the future of the arts in healthcare.

As I conclude this book, I reflect on the challenges of performing in paediatrics in a post-pandemic era. I also address questions about changing the ways arts can support hospitalised children by recognising and valuing the difference between staying true to yourself as an actor, acting in harmony with who you are and what you believe, valuing your 'insides', your feelings and beliefs, and match your 'insides' with your actions and being realistic when once works in healthcare. It is essential to explore whether arts-based activities can support hospitalised children and their relevance to possible scenarios for how the arts for health will adapt and react to future pandemics or epidemic crises. By looking at the rising need for alternative ways of delivering the arts on hospital wards, actors are challenged to explore strategies for adaptation while maintaining synergies of stories and emotions with audiences at the core of their applied theatre practice. Cziboly and Bethlenfalvy (2020) present ways of facilitating process dramas online by using planning, facilitation, telling a story, framing, distancing, protection, conventions and Teacher-in-Role. My experience of transferring physical bedside performances to digital platforms so that my projects could continue supporting children in hospitals during the COVID-19 pandemic was challenging because new skills and strategies had to be employed in a minimal schedule. I had to react to the chaos caused by the crisis and respond swiftly to my projects' actors, hospitals and funders with creative proposals. Despite the focus on surviving the difficulties, the challenge was also exciting. In many ways, this deceivingly simple practice of performing live on digital platforms and accessing children on their teachers' devices constitutes a political act. I began to recognise a demand for outreaching children during a global and personal crisis and performance as a valuable form of joy and relaxation. We had to be creative and introduce new ways of overcoming technical problems and making new meanings of the art form and its possibilities beyond traditional theatre uses.

The experience of 'Rocket-Arts' has revealed that setting live bedside participatory performances and digital films on the wards against one another is misplaced. The AEA report Consulting for the Arts Council of England 'From live-to-digital' Report offers an overview of the shift between live performance to broadcasted performance and insight into digital developments in theatre on audiences, production and distribution. The report recasts notions of live and non-live performance to argue:

> *The focus should be placed on how England's theatre sector can remain vibrant, vital, and relevant while embracing both Live-to-Digital and live. Live-to-Digital signals neither the death nor the salvation of live theatre. Rather, it represents one means of harnessing rapidly evolving technologies and audience expectations to widen the scope of live theatrical performance. Live-to-Digital cannot replace the individual live performance that remains the core of theatre's unique appeal; nor is anyone trying to do this. Instead, it offers a means by which certain performances can be experienced by more audiences, particularly younger and more diverse ones, in new ways, and it should take its place as one element in theatre's ever-evolving relationship with its audience. It is not the whole future, but it is here to stay and may very well be an essential element of long-term success for theatre organisations in England, both on and off the stage.*
>
> (AEA 2016, p. 16)

So, while I was reading the report, I realised it was visionary because it paved the way for rapid developments in digital evolution in the theatre industry without even knowing what was yet to come due to the COVID-19 pandemic. Although I rarely have an opportunity to discuss if or how technology results in lasting goals around health and wellbeing in conjunction with the arts, I know that something significant happened during the pandemic, and it is still happening through a creative process of marrying live performance with the digital so that the arts become accessible to children and their families during their stay in the hospital. Moreover, arts-based projects contribute to possibilities for a better quality of care, a vision and a must of healthcare providers and alternative ways of being and living at times of negativity, difficulty and vulnerability. Children can participate in activities inspired by the arts as stimuli and gain opportunities to create and share their throughs and emotions with their caregivers and healthcare professionals.

In reflection, it would be unwise to ignore that the 'Rocket-Arts' experience has raised some serious questions for me:

- How are hospitals responding to the availability of new digital projects for their patients?
- How do the overpowering trends in digital arts impact the need to protect live performance's artistic and cultural integrity in paediatrics?
- Is consumption of digital projects in paediatrics being achieved at the expense of participation in synergistic performance events on hospital wards?
- Can the language of care be developed through animation at the same standards as it can be established through intimate performance?
- What is driving the arts in healthcare profession: is it persistence in physical participatory bedside performance, or is the availability of new media for the provision of the arts in healthcare stimulating a hidden necessity?

- Which future combinations of bedside live performance and digital technology are most appropriate for children in hospitals in this context?
- How can we envisage which future projects are most appropriate for sick children and plan strategically for their design and implementation?
- How can we share information about arts-based cooperative productions with healthcare and medical professionals?

To explore synergies between art and technology in applied theatre practice in paediatrics, we need to remember a distinction vital to understanding arts-based interventions: the physical and the non-physical, the face-to-face participation and the digital interaction, the intimate and the animate. New technologies and media for storytelling in participatory forms may help us study how children's minds perceive and understand the difference between performing arts and digital arts. Boyd (2009) argues that the domains of intimate and animate in stories bring different expectations and draw on other inferences from physiology and psychology about art, religion and rituality. In this sense, stories don't impose outcomes and fixed endings on audiences but cause audiences to use their feelings for witnessing, feeling and responding in their ways. It is not in the focus of this book to investigate the complicated connection between body and brain and cognitive, mental, emotional and spiritual understandings of the world. However, I see the moment as an opportunity to start thinking of creating a model where theatre practitioners and digital artists consider both intimacy and animation, physicality and psychology, cognition and spirituality as aspects of the art form to pursue artistic work at the highest level outside of stereotypical work models. Such a model honours the interplay of creativity, cooperation, co-imagination, co-experience and co-narration in a language that does not fall into narrow and fundamentalistic representations of life events. This work requires internal awareness and mental representation of events that children experience in hospitals and events that we witness and recreate through imagination to create a narrative that the children could relate to. Such a model will require comprehending children's experiences. Still, we cannot represent or entirely understand all of their ill health-related experiences even if we employ technological and creative inventiveness. The 'Rocket-Arts' project taught me that. Therefore, there remains a persistent gap in knowledge and analysis around the functions and benefits of applied theatre emerging models for sick children in healthcare settings. Alrutz (2015) argues that digital and performance-based approaches offer opportunities to explore the relationships between identity, experience and power, engaging young people and developing both young people and actors' understanding of power and learning. Before we understand the inherent opportunities in digital art technology, I am sharing some questions with the reader to help me explore the collaboration possibilities in practice.

- How can we invite actors to acknowledge the differences between intimate performance on the hospital wards and remote digital facilitation of artistic work?

- How can we invite healthcare professionals to support digital arts-based practices with hospitalised children without actors on the wards until the restrictions for artists visiting hospitals are lifted?
- Is it acceptable for nurses and hospital teachers to work as 'substitutes' for arts facilitators in the absence of artists on hospital wards during the pandemic? What training will that work require?
- How can digital arts and storytelling work disrupt biased approaches to ill children's ability and ownership of stories?
- How can healthcare systems embrace and support change in the delivery of the arts in paediatrics by visualising creative spaces in hospitals where children, families and staff can engage and experience combinations of art forms, media and applications?
- How can actors and healthcare professionals collaborate to make the need for upgraded systems of support for the arts in hospitals visible to clinical management teams and decision-makers?
- How can artists with patients, service users and healthcare professionals become involved throughout arts-based research projects (e.g. reviewing the aims, developing the digital tools/materials, supporting the ethics application, advising on the questions, recruitment plans, etc., disseminating the findings)?
- What new pedagogical frameworks and models can we create around learning about applied arts in health that value collaborative efforts and acknowledge the importance of artistic quality and property?
- And, how can artists train healthcare professionals to consider the intellectual property generated by actors within collaborative projects between clinical staff and arts-based facilitators and researchers?
- What strategic planning can artists make to challenge traditional power dynamics between actors and healthcare professionals in research about the impact of the arts on children's health in clinical contexts and settings?
- How can artists create inter-disciplinary communities of performers, film producers, and technical and clinical staff in healthcare to develop hybrid arts-based practices for broader groups of young patients?
- How can researchers further investigate the relationship between caring for the audience in healthcare and emotional labour (e.g. how artists express and communicate emotions in clinical settings, defining what emotions artists experience, and the degree to which artists' feelings are observed, processed and managed)?

Raising the above questions from a theoretical and practical perspective constitutes political with a small 'p', a need to improve how applied arts in paediatrics and healthcare are generally formed, executed, evaluated and valued. The constant work of working in partnership with healthcare requires attention to this question – the politics of arts for health and passion and determination. Providing opportunities for producing knowledge and viable arts-based practices in paediatrics requires reforms in the mentality of both actors and healthcare professionals and close collaboration between the two professions.

This work requires a reformation in educational provision for actors. First, the training courses for actors should gradually consider the arts for children and young people in health and community care systems as 'relevant' for study and discussion in drama training courses. For example, acting, characterisation, vocalisation, improvisation, communication and critical thinking are skills that should be, in my view, considered as closely related to everyday situations actors face in hospitals. The stories that I discussed in this book demonstrate that it is possible that actors can use these skills to approach and communicate with children, to understand children's emotional needs better, and by doing that, enable healthcare professionals to assess pain and offer children the proper care. And yet, the choice of content for educational drama provision usually reflects providers' educational policy and educational standing regarding what is appropriate for the actor's profession. Higher education systems, as the situation in the UK demonstrates, can also be 'political footballs', kicked around by changing political parties without trying to stay neutral and consistent with society's needs. Thus, universities and colleges need to fight for the arts to engage with actors in a movement towards possibility, new methods and better conditions for arts to improve individual and community health and wellbeing. Additional critical inquiries are needed to provide evidence about the influence of applied arts on children's emotions on audiences in less ordinary settings such as hospitals when routines of normality and supporting networks collapse during the COVID-19 pandemic. As part of my reflection on these changes, I think there will be a further impact on the need for combined mixed-approach and mixed-media, 'hybrid' arts-based interventions in healthcare, but lack of funding will also heighten the challenges.

Pragmatically, at the moment, a crucial problem facing the integration of arts-based practice in healthcare in the UK is that there is a declining governmental commitment to fund the arts. While the UK government announced £260 million to boost healthcare research and manufacturing for the period 2021–2024 (GOV. UK 2022), the arts are, once more, intimidated, destabilised and threatened, which is a potential avenue for further research around the political will for the sustainability of the arts in healthcare. Some previous examples of art interventions in hospitals were supplemented with money from local charitable trusts. Short funds provide the actors with no assurance that arts in healthcare will be sustained. To be realistic, actors cannot wait for continued state funding to come. However, this is not to argue that there is a situation where there must be government support or no arts in paediatrics. Despite and beyond economics, I say that it becomes necessary to fund the arts for all its benefits for the patients. Furthermore, recognising the value of the difference between cultures, language, media, forms and practices will be challenging. Still, it could also provide an opportunity for a shift in perception of the arts in times of crisis as a valuable and essential tool to build more robust models for efficient health and community care.

Understandably, the pandemic spread pessimism and caused anxiety amongst actors about the absence of arts-based projects in healthcare for over two years of unemployment. It also imposed the production of alternative artistic creations such as live-streamed performances, films, apps and online resources. Ultimately, community actors and arts organisations focused on children and the potential of using technology to create new possibilities. Sharing stories online and inviting children to engage with characters in films and other digital media constitutes an essential step in delivering arts in healthcare that disturbs and disrupts traditional face-to-face bedside performance promises for new possibilities. Still, questions about artistic values and priorities are also valid. Actors working to support children in hospitals must be willing to look at and examine their roles, skills and responsibilities as actors in healthcare. Specifically, actors using the art form to build a performer–audience relationship based on empathy and compassion rather than pure entertainment must be willing to protect and preserve the work's aesthetics.

The future of the arts is unknown in the light of constant cuts in funding; it is up to individual motivation based on evidence about the value of the arts in healthcare to propose creative solutions and ways in which we can use a passion for artistic practice as well as our compassion for vulnerable children, to help them. More needs to be done in paediatrics to withstand the changes of the pandemic crisis and move forward. There is a need to respond to the needs of children, families and the healthcare professionals who work with them, hear their opinions about the healthcare systems that just started recovering after the covid and find allies in a battle with challenge and unpredictability.

Time for change

In my view, the case for change in the provision of the participatory arts in healthcare is vital, and the need for action is critical. The future of applied theatre forms and practices in paediatrics is changing in response to the demands of our times. We must think, plan and adapt if we are serious about keeping up with the developments in societies, healthcare systems and the creative arts industry. We must be serious about preparing sick children to overcome the challenging aspects of hospitalisation through the arts. In that case, we must train artists to perform confidently, sensitively and wisely in the children's hospital world.

I began this book by welcoming the power of stories in participatory theatre for sick children and a personal commitment to normalising the hospital experience. I argue that there are essential priorities if the arts are to meet the many challenges that healthcare systems now face because of the COVID-19 pandemic crisis. I tried to define my understanding of the role of participatory arts in healthcare, the opportunities and problems in current provision as we see them and as they have been presented to us through artists in healthcare and hospital teachers through research and consultations. There is a need for balance in the policy about the arts in health or about health through the arts, in the structure of the provision of the arts in hospitals, in training methods of the artist and the healthcare professional, in the assessment of the quality of practice, in the partnerships and relationships between arts organisations, theatre companies, freelance artists and hospital staff, ward managers and agencies, and in the training of people. We need to think through the implications in principle and practice of a genuine commitment of people, organisations, health providers and cultural agencies to realise the potential of participatory theatre for children in hospitals and improve their wellbeing in tough times. I also shared my research about artists' and healthcare professionals' emotional and professional needs working with vulnerable children to realise their creative potential of developing their cross-disciplinary knowledge and understanding. Promoting cross-disciplinary innovative education is complex because it will involve a study of the two cultures, for example, theatre and nursing, and a review of styles of work, purposes and ethos of various professions. I believe that this will require time and dedication. I also think that this is a must, not an option.

To ensure that applied theatre in healthcare has a sustainable future in finances and infrastructure and that the importance of training on arts and health is recognised and provided in higher education and colleges, I raise some recommendations for actions by healthcare providers, governments and artists. These proposals are personal based on my experience of applied theatre for children and young people in healthcare and education in England, Europe and Australia for the past 30 years. Substantial reports about arts and health have offered me a range of projects as examples, perspectives and recommendations. Amongst these are the All-Party Parliamentary Group Creative Health Report (2017) and the World Health Organisation scoping review about the role of the arts in improving health and wellbeing (Fancourt & Finn 2019). In these reports, arts and science offer examples of creativity in complementary ways. Although declarations about the arts for health didn't find new cures for children's cancer, they launched a thousand opportunities for growing the arts' capacity to secure attention, foster cooperation and raise awareness about its contribution to health and wellbeing. Still, despite knowing that the arts appeal to human growth and happiness, science has to account for healthcare systems not created to suit the arts or artistic talents.

Although the arts are precious and speak to many, they are often treated as the icing on the case of healthcare provision. For a constant condition of the arts embedded in healthcare services during hospitalisation, we must disturb the traditional notions of hospitals as medical territories by producing evidence-based non-pharmaceutical approaches to illness. One of the challenges in England today is that healthcare is becoming a shared enterprise and will become a collaborative provision. It will be provided not only by hospitals and general practices but by businesses, commercial organisations and professionals in technology, robotics and society. Promoting the arts for health and enhancing healthcare through the arts is more imperative than ever. The arts must be invited to lend their expertise, resources and experience in healthcare's changing landscape. For that reason, healthcare providers and governments are mainly responsible for creating and further improving those pathways of collaboration between the arts and healthcare. That is because they are the ones who approve or refuse partnerships with arts organisations and practitioners based on financial terms and subject-specific priorities. What a world this can be! Understanding the borders between arts and health in pursuing collaborations and new projects has been challenging. Still, the experience of bringing the arts into the hospital wards at times of financial and social ambiguity inspires me for more action. The recommendations of actions by healthcare professionals and governments in this chapter aim to move things forward by engaging those who make decisions about the provision of the arts in clinical settings.

In writing recommendations for actions that appeal to the reader's intelligence, I recalled the 'All Our Futures' (NACCCE Report 1999) and its contribution to unlocking children's creativity in the English national curriculum. The NACCCE report continues to enthuse me today in how it puts the case for developing a national creative and cultural education strategy. It is still relevant because it looks for connections between people's capacities for original ideas and action, people's engagement with the complexity of practice and ways of learning and the partnerships between organisations and the wider world. I take the opportunity to argue that intellectual and practical differences may be tied to the ethos of each discipline (education versus healthcare) and the era between now and then. But my assumption remains that there are meaningful relationships between the arts and healthcare and significant implications for methods of teaching and implementation as there were between the arts and education 20 years ago. I am aware that these recommendations cannot all apply to all cultural and healthcare systems and that they cannot be implemented immediately. However, some of them call for immediate action. The best we can do is to create opportunities for artists and healthcare professionals to work together for the benefit of sick children, to develop the capacities of both professionals as fully as possible so that they will be equipped for whatever pandemic or epidemic crises do face in the future.

Actions by healthcare providers

- Healthcare providers and governments should raise the priority they give to children's health and wellbeing; promote the management of hospital experiences and encourage the participation of children and young people in the co-production and co-design of arts projects in healthcare.
- The development plans of children's hospitals need to be more explicitly connected to the provision of arts for sick children and their families during hospitalisation, including the provision of bedside performances and digital interventions; the opportunities to meet and work with professional artists, not artists-in-residence necessarily, and with specialists and cultural organisations from outside the healthcare systems.
- Hospitals should explore practical ways of embedding arts-based projects in their facilities to enrich the experience of children and their families during treatment.
- Healthcare providers must develop their capacity to ensure that expert advice and consultation are offered to artists in healthcare on specialist areas of hospital life and routines, safeguarding policies and training, healthcare provision and standards.
- Hospital arts managers need to be appointed to coordinate the provision of arts in hospitals and conduct an audit of the quality of projects for all the

children-patients, including opportunities for interactive participation through creative and imaginative media.
- Healthcare plans for hospital staff who work with children, such as nurses and doctors, should include a provision to improve hospital staff's understanding of the arts and the benefits of bedside participatory arts for their patients. Knowledge and experience may facilitate better collaborations between artists and hospital staff.
- The paediatric arts services should be available to all children and their families based on equality, diversity, inclusion and equity. To this end, there should be a greater emphasis in hospitals on arts provision for all.

Actions by local authorities and governments

- Local authorities in association with the government should provide arts organisations with dedicated funds for arts-based projects and activities for children in healthcare and enable them to coordinate the provision of the arts in hospital settings and contexts.
- Local authorities in association with the government should provide research institutes with dedicated funds for arts-based projects and activities for children in healthcare and enable them to evaluate the provision of the arts in hospital settings and contexts.
- Local authorities, in association with the government, should establish a sustainable system for long-term funding for the arts in child healthcare. Ad hoc funds are helpful but cannot secure the sustainability of practice and its benefits for sick children.
- Local authorities and governments should allocate core funds to the progression of long-lasting partnerships between arts and healthcare providers and organisations to ensure that the arts provision in healthcare is embedded in healthcare. Informal, sporadic, scattered and occasional provision of the arts in healthcare needs to become constant, steady, and centred on supporting long-term and short-term patients.
- The government should also encourage and fund arts-based projects for hospitalised children. The goal should be to offer each child at least one arts-based project during their hospitalisation and provide resources and materials to ensure that all children in hospitals have had opportunities to experience the participatory arts.

Actions by artists

- Artists and arts organisations should aim for high-quality projects for vulnerable children and their families. Artistic interventions should all contribute to improving children's health and wellbeing.
- Artists and arts organisations should aim for high-quality projects for vulnerable children and their families. They should undertake systematic and rigorous evaluation of their work, including existing training, techniques,

methods of artistry and skills to develop realistic understandings of their practice, the strengths and weaknesses of the work and plan strategically to make improvements.
- Based on widening participation, professionally trained artists from various cultural backgrounds should be encouraged to collaborate with healthcare providers, provided that a safe, ethical and constructive collaboration between artists and healthcare professionals is secured. That is to ensure diversity and inclusion in the provision of the arts in healthcare and to create opportunities for children from various ethnic and cultural backgrounds to participate in projects they can relate to.
- The value of artistic work in healthcare should be prioritised by ensuring that artists have the freedom to devise arts projects to meet the requirements of artistic excellence.
- Arts organisations interested in working with sick children should develop policies related to health and wellbeing. Such policies should not impose healthcare priorities on the artistic work's objectives but should recognise the need to engage with healthcare as an objective. Instead, such policies should guide artists on dealing with challenging situations in healthcare environments and how working in challenging settings will impact the artist's performance and wellbeing.
- Arts organisations interested in working with sick children should be creating opportunities for their members to discuss their training needs on both professional skills and emotional competencies, the full implications of performing to vulnerable audiences and encourage them to respond to the challenges of the work in formal and informal ways.
- Given the circumstances created during the COVID-19 pandemic regarding the demand to work with hospitalised children remotely by using technology, arts organisations should explore creative uses of technology.

I have argued that the provision of the arts in healthcare needs to further improve in England, possibly elsewhere in the world. Part of the problem with the provision of arts in child healthcare is that healthcare systems focus on traditional medical and pharmaceutical treatments and have a limited understanding of the benefits of participatory arts for children's health and wellbeing. This situation underestimates a large part of the scope, potential and efficacy of the arts, creating the time and the space to think, dream and improve lives. Suppose societies are to develop seriously caring support systems for children as humans, not only as patients or pupils. In that case, we must also first acknowledge how rich and diverse the artistic resources are. Outside hospitals, the arts are recognised as entertainment and education, evident in the richness of creative events and learning programmes. A more balanced healthcare system must provide opportunities for the arts to play an instrumental part in healthcare during treatment and recovery. A more human stay during hospitalisation should provide opportunities for all sick and injured children to experience the arts, or aspects of it, through a holistic healthcare approach to illness and cure. Applied theatre in paediatrics is not a diversion from the healthcare medical provision. It is an essential tool for making meaning of illness, putting it into a fictional context, and developing better control of their clinical experiences. Applied theatre in paediatrics can be central to raising the standards of care and quality of life during illness.

So, I will insist on finding creative, efficient and sustainable ways of applying theatre to hospitalised children. These are children who are anxious before and after surgery, children who experience life-threatening conditions, children who are on medication and experience side effects that affect their being, children who visit hospitals for routine treatments, and children who spend more time in hospital than in their bedrooms, children who have all the care they deserve and others who experience neglect and abuse, children who are blessed with a loving family and children whose families are scattered or unknown, children with supportive environments and others who rely on the healthcare and social care system for support, children who feel secure in their cultural identities and children who are scared and feel sad by living in new places away from home, children who have friends waiting for them in school and children who are alone. The children I will continue working for are poor and rich, children of all races, genders, cultures, social and economic backgrounds, and children of the world who are ill and undergoing treatment. And their parents and families too. In fear and trembling, in excitement and cautiousness, I recall the hours when children's suffering in hospital became mine, and in times of reflection in solitude, I pray for those children as if they are mine.

References

AEA Consulting for Arts Council England, UK Theatre and Society of London Theatre 2016, *From love-to-digital. Understanding the impact of digital developments in theatre on audiences, production, and distribution*. www.artscouncil.org.uk/sites/default/files/download-file/From_Live_to_Digital_OCT2016.pdf.

All-Party Parliamentary Group 2017, Creative health: The arts for health and wellbeing. *APPG*. www.culturehealthandwellbeing.org.uk/appg-inquiry/Publications/Creative_Health_Inquiry_Report_2017_-_Second_Edition.pdf.

Alrutz, M 2015, *Digital Storytelling, Applied Theatre, & Youth Performing Possibility*, Routledge: London.

Boyd, B 2009, *On the Origin of Stories. Evolution, Cognition and Fiction*, The Belknap Press of Harvard University: Cambridge, MA.

Conlon, C, McDonnell, T, Barrett, Ml, Cummins, F, Deasy, C, Hensey, C, McAuliffe, E & Nicholson, E 2021, 'The impact of the COVID-19 pandemic on child health and the provision of Care in paediatric emergency departments: A qualitative study of frontline emergency care staff', *BMC Health Services Research*, vol. 21, no. 279. https://pubmed.ncbi.nlm.nih.gov/33766026/.

Cziboly, A & Bethlenfalvy, B 2020, 'Response to COVID-19 zooming in on online process drama', *Research in Drama Education: The Journal of Applied Theatre and Performance*. www.researchgate.net/publication/344256873_Response_to_COVID-19_Zooming_in_on_online_process_drama.

Fancourt, D & Finn, S 2019, *What is the Evidence on the Role of the Arts in Improving Health and Well-being? A Scoping Review* (Health Evidence Network synthesis report, no. 67), World Health Organisation: Copenhagen.

GOV. UK 2022, *Press Release £260 million to boost healthcare research and manufacturing*. www.gov.uk/government/news/260-million-to-boost-healthcare-research-and-manufacturing.

Mak, HW, Fluharty, MF & Fancourt, D 2021, 'Predictors and impact of arts engagement during the COVID-19 pandemic: Analyses of data from 19,384 adults in the COVID-19 social study', *Frontiers in Psychology*. https://doi.org/10.3389/fpsyg.2021.626263.

Meherali, S, Punjani, N, Louie-Poon, S, Rahim, KA, Das, JK, Salam, RA & Lassi, ZS 2021, 'Mental health of children and adolescents amidst COVID-19 and past pandemics: A rapid systematic review', *International Journal of Environmental Research and Public Health*, vol. 18, no. 7. https://doi.org/10.3390/ijerph18073432.

National Advisory Committee on Creative and Cultural Education, NACCCE 1999, *All our futures report. Creativity, culture and education*. https://sirkenrobinson.com/pdf/allourfutures.pdf.

Prior, R 2020, 'Training the animator a new: Developing cross-disciplinary opportunities for puppetry in arts, health and education', *Journal of Applied Arts & Health*, vol. 11, no. 1–2, pp. 73–83.

Racine, N, Cooke, JE, Eirich, R, Korczak, DJ, McArthur, B & Madigan, S 2020, 'Child and adolescent mental illness during COVID-19: A rapid review', *Psychiatry Research*, vol. 292. https://pubmed.ncbi.nlm.nih.gov/32707216/.

Singh, S, Roy, D, Sinha, K, Parveen, S, Sharma, G & Joshi, G 2020, 'Impact of COVID-19 and lockdown on mental health of children and adolescents: A narrative review with recommendations', *Psychiatry Research*, vol. 293. https://doi.org/10.1016/j.psychres.2020.113429.

The Children's Society 2021, *The Impact of COVID-19 on Children and Young People*, London. www.childrenssociety.org.uk/sites/default/files/2021-01/the-impact-of-COVID-19-on-children-and-young-people-briefing.pdf.

APPENDIX A

'Rocket-Arts' or Simba, the therapy dog. The script

Persephone Sextou

I wrote this story inspired by our family cocker spaniel named Simba. Simba's breed is very energetic and boisterous, curious and excitable. Not many cockers are trained as therapy dogs for that reason. Using a Labrador as a calm and well-behaved dog in hospitals would have been more realistic. But, the love and affection that Simba gives to our family inspired me to make him the story's character. Simba has been there for all of us during the COVID-19 pandemic. Simba has been loyal, friendly, caring and present for good and bad times. So there you have Simba, a lively dog helping an ill child escape the hospital walls and fly to space in their imagination.

> Simba is a therapy dog.
> A therapy dog is a dog that is trained to provide affection, comfort and love to children in hospitals.
> Simba is an adorable golden Labrador with big brown friendly eyes and a lovely temperament.
> He works at the children's hospital with his trainer Lucy.
> Simba wears a yellow vest saying 'I am here for you' and his volunteer budge with his picture.
> He is so smart! He knows it's time to go to work when he puts on his vest in the morning.
> Days are busy for Simba, but he never complains.
> A treat or two, and he is good. Life on the wards is full of smiles, giggles, wagging tails, cuddles, kisses and fun when Simba is around.
> It is Tuesday evening, and Simba is visiting Tom.
> Tom has video monitoring in his bed tomorrow.
> The doctors want to see on the screen how his brain works.

He has to wash his hair tonight to get ready for tomorrow.
Tom knows they will attach tiny metal pieces with some sticky glue to his head.
Mum says, 'it will be as sticky as your fingers when you have pancakes with syrup!'
Tom laughed. He loves pancakes with syrup!
Wednesday morning.

Dr Phillips entered the room and went next to Tom's bed.

Dr Phillips: Hi Tom, I am Doctor Fillip, and I am here today to do some screening. This will help us to see how your brain works. OK?

Tom keeps quiet and drifts closer to his mum.

Dr Phillips: I hear that you like stories. Is that true?

Tom is nodding.

Dr Phillips: I knew it! Let me guess. Do you like watching the stars?

Tom is nodding.

Dr Phillips: Would you like to join Simba in lifting off his spaceship to explore a galaxy? Your head must be full of images of astronauts ready to lift off their spaceship to explore our universe. Is that so?

Tom is nodding again.

Dr Phillips: I used to love space stories when I was your age. I would be privileged if you let me scan some of those space images. Would that be ok?

Tom's heart is going fast now. He is panting.

Tom's mum: Are you ok, honey?
Tom: I am scared. He hides his face with the pillow and starts crying.
Dr Phillips: It's ok, Tom. It's ok to cry. The nurse will look after you. I will be back tomorrow. The doctor smiles and leaves the room.

At that moment, Simba popped into the room.

Tom's mum: Look who is here!

A smile spreads across Tom's face.

Tom: Simba! You are here!

Tom wipes his tears with his hand and giggles to replace his fear.
Simba goes closer to Tom for a treat. Mum squirts cheese on Tom's hand for Simba to lick. He is licking Tom's hand, sharing love and affection.

Lucy: Simba loves cheese.

Tom gives Simba a big cuddle, and Simba wags his tail happily.

Tom: Can I stroke him today? Please!?
Lucy: All right then.

Tom reaches out, grasps the brush and slowly strokes Simba's coat.

Tom: Look, mum, Simba loves it.

Tom is smiling and breathing normally. He is just fine.

Tom: I am so glad you are here, Simba.
Lucy: Simba needs some rest now. See you later, Tom.
Tom: Could Simba be here for the screen monitoring tomorrow when the doctor comes?

Lucy has to ask the nurses if that would be possible. She promises to come back tomorrow with an answer.
It is Thursday morning.
Tom is getting ready to have his video monitoring in his bed.
Doctor Fillip wants to see how his brain works.

Dr Phillips: Hi Tom, How are you feeling today?

Tom is quiet.
He is looking at the door, hoping Simba will show up, but there is no sign of Simba yet.
Tom is thinking, 'Where are you, Simba? I can't go through this without you'.

Dr Philip: I am here to examine you, Tom. Are you ready?

Tom's waiting for Simba.
His heart is beating like a jungle drum.
Tom is panting. He is scared.
He wants to run away, but he can't.
Before he knows it, a familiar figure appears at the door.

Tom: Simba! You are here!

Tom opens his arms, and Simba goes near his bed with confidence.

Tom: Can he stay with me? Please?
Dr Phillips: OK then. I will let him stay in the room if he is still calm.

Lucy promises that Simba will be as still and calm as a statue.

Dr Philip: Are you ready to begin?

Tom looks at Simba's big brown mesmerising eyes and feels reassured and relaxed.

Tom: Yes, I am ready.

While Dr Phillips starts the procedure, Simba stays still on his back legs and watches Tom.
Their eyes meet each other.
Simba and Tom are connecting.
Instant connection.
Something magical is happening.
Different.
Tom sees Simba's eyes becoming screens just like his computer screen.

Tom: Wow! It is like a video game! How do you do this, Simba?
Dr Phillips: Stay calm, Tom. You are doing well.

Tom is drawstring.
He falls fast asleep.
He is dreaming.
In his dream, he sees colourful images of stars and galaxies.
Simba: Ready to land off?
Tom and Simba fly in space.
They see the Earth from space.
It is a tiny, blue dot.
It is so beautiful.
Their spaceship is off to the Moon.
They have arrived on the moon.
Simba is wearing a space suit and sits next to Tom.
They are on a spacecraft off to a distant planet.
They see flashing comets with long sparkling tails passing by.
They see the Earth from space. It is a tiny, blue dot. It is so beautiful.
Next, they are behind the dark side of the moon.

Millions of stars are ahead of them.
Before they know it, they face a bright red planet like a giant dragon eye.
They were in the middle of a space dust storm.
Tom and Simba turn around Mars and enter a space dust storm.
Their spacecraft is sailing amongst shiny little stars glittering like jewellery.

Dr Phillips: Your mind is in motion.

Tom can't hear him. His mind is miles away in animated milky galaxies.

Dr Phillips: It is all over now. Hold on a minute. What's this on the screen?

Dr Fillip points to a bright object in a fast motion on the screen.
He looks closer and jumps up from his chair.

Dr Phillips: It's a space rocket!

Everyone in the room laughed.
Simba blinked his eyes and barked happily.
Lucy gave him a treat, and Tom woke up.
Mum kissed Tom on his cheek.
Dr Phillip congratulates Tom.

Dr Phillips: Well done, young man. Or should I say, young spaceman?

Dr Phillips winked to Simba.
Simba wagged his tail to wink back.

Tom: Thank you, Dr Phillips.
Dr Phillips: You are the bravest boy I have met, Tom.

Simba barks enthusiastically.
Dr Phillip offers his hand in the high-five position and waits for Simba to paw his open palm.
Simba high-fives his hand and gets his reward, a tasty treat.

Lucy: Good boy, Simba. Good boy!

When Tom is in hospital feeling worried, and his heart is running fast, Simba, the therapy dog, is there to absorb his fears like a sponge and help him be brave. After all, that's what good friends are for.

APPENDIX B

'Lollie the rough collie and the magic kiss'.
The story

Persephone Sextou

If I had a dog, it would be a rough collie dog. My mother had one, and my great-grandfather had one. If I had a dog, it would be a large, slim, intelligent dog like my mother's. It would have arched eyebrows and dark almond-shaped eyes like my grandfather's dog. It would have a white and brown coat with a long tail with a twist like my great grandfather's dog. My dog would be the most beautiful. I would call her Lollie, my adorable rough collie!

I think about this dog when I am in the hospital. When the lights are off in the ward, and I can see no stars in the night sky out of the window, Lollie comes into my dreams, and we go on adventures.

Together, we play and laugh and dance and bark, and together we are happy. We don't eat the same food, but we have many lollies. We don't have the same age, but we have the same hobbies. We don't speak the same language, but we like playing with dollies. When I say to her 'stop', she would stop, when I tell her 'sit', she would sit, and when I say to her 'up', she would stand up on her back feet and lick my face.

In my dreams, we walk on the seaside and run after the seagulls. We race and fall and get covered with sand. We see the fishers putting out fish nets on their boats in the morning. We see the sun setting on a pillow of orange and purple colours in the evening. Our last stop is the sweet little shop. Lollie and I always treat ourselves with a ball of the most delicious ice cream.

One night I dreamt we were on my grandfather's farm. My grandfather lives on a farm filled with cherry trees. It is a paradise in the spring. The cherry blossoms bloom in spring, and they are heavenly and breath-taking. The trees show off their flowers when the skies are clear and the sun is bright. When the wind blows, the petals dance in the air like ballerinas. That night I dreamt I visited the farm with Lollie.

It was a sunny morning. My grandfather was waiting for us at the gate. We walked to the field at the back of the house. He asked if we were ready to see the most beautiful scene. He pointed to the cherry trees. The trees were covered in pink petals, and busy bees were buzzing, saying, 'spring is here!' We admired the pink colours, and we smelled the scent.

Lollie was excited! She kept jumping and hopping. She was rolling in the grass and rubbing her neck and back on my grandfather's boots. She looked so happy to me, but my grandfather said that Lollie was behaving strangely and that he hadn't seen her being so weird for weeks. One moment she was jumping and stretching; the next, she dropped to the ground making an impression of a corpse. My grandfather said, 'I am going to fetch her ball from the shed,' and disappeared behind the truck. Lollie and I were left alone.

I didn't know what to do with her. I told her to 'stop', but she wouldn't stop. I told her to 'sit', but she wouldn't sit. I told her to stand 'up,' but she ignored me completely. Lollie started jumping around. She was out of control. She ran away from me in the field where I could not see her anymore. I called out her name many times with no reply. I whistled, but still nothing. Suddenly I felt alone. The sky turned grey, and the cherry petals fell from the trees. I climbed to the top of a tree to look for Lollie. No sign of her. The world seemed empty without her.

The following day I asked my mum if she had ever had a bad experience with her dog. She told me a story. She said that her dog was once stung by a swarm of bees, and she had to take him to the vet. It was really painful for her dog. The vet said that he had never seen a dog stung so many times and that the dog had an allergic reaction to the stings. Mum said his face was swollen, and he had problems with breathing, but the vet pulled out the sting, gave him a syrup, and looked after him. She bathed him in soda and water and applied ice packs on his nose every 5 minutes to reduce the swelling. He was fine after a couple of days.

Mum smiled and told me that dogs have feelings like us, and sometimes they know how we feel. They suffer from pain as people do, and they recover with love. We don't understand it, but it's good to remember it. She kissed me goodnight and took a seat next to me. I wish I were in my grandfather's field. I wish I could see the stars glimmering. Like the other night, I dreamt of Lollie, my adorable rough collie.

I was in the middle of the cherry farm looking for Lollie. At that moment, I thought I saw something moving behind the trees. It was not clear at first, but it was her! Lollie! I ran to her with my arms open, calling her name, Lollie! It's you! It was her, but, 'Oh no!' Her face was all swollen up! Her mouth and nose had doubled in size! I took her in my arms. 'What happened to you, girl?' 'Are you stung?' 'Were you playing with the bees?' I asked her. She looked at me sheepishly. She was scratching her nose to let me know that something was wrong with it. She wouldn't let me touch her nose, but I could tell it wasn't good. She wasn't jumping up and down anymore. She laid flat on one side and looked at me. A teardrop fell from her eye down on my hand. 'Lollie, are you crying? I didn't know dogs could cry! Oh, Lollie!' I remember that teardrop on my hand. It looked like a pearl tattoo. And then, she closed her eyes. I panicked.

'Lollie, wake up! Please!' I was so scared. Lollie, my rough collie, is the most beautiful of all dogs because she is mine. Lollie, my rough collie, is the most precious of all dogs because she is my friend. Lollie, my rough collie, is in pain. I looked around, seeking my grandfather, but I was alone with a suffering dog under an old cherry tree. And then I heard a voice saying, 'Remember, dogs have feelings. They suffer from pain and recover with love as people do.'

Suddenly I felt strong. 'That's it.' I thought. 'I know what to do. I will show her that I love her.' My dog needed me. I was not a baby anymore. I was big enough to look after her.

I was brave enough not to let her suffer. I was strong enough to take good care of her and tell her not to be afraid. I didn't worry anymore. I searched for the sting. It was like a small black needle. I pinched it from her skin with my fingers.

'All I can do is love you', I whispered to her ear and gave her a warm, adoring kiss. Nothing happened for a moment or two, but the sun came out, the cherry blossom scent filled the air, and the trees around us showed off their bright colours again in full spring blossom. Pink petals fell on Lollie's nose just where the sting was. I looked up at the sky, and the petals were dancing like ballerinas above us. It was a magical moment.

Lollie opened her eyes, sneezed, and stood up. She barked happily and licked my face like a lollypop enthusiastically. That was some kiss! I knew that she was letting me know she loved me. Her face looked just fine. It was back to normal. She was her good old self again. She was jumping and hopping around. 'I love you, Lollie!'

The following day, there was a cherry petal on my pillow. I stretched my hand to touch it and saw the most fantastic thing. A pearl drop was marked on my skin. 'Lollie's tear!' I said a tattoo reminds me that love is the best of all remedies and cures everything.' Love makes cherry trees blossom.

INDEX

aesthetic(s) 15, 26, 29, 86, 90; aesthetic distance 6, 54, 87–88; aesthetic experience 34, 99–100
agency (during performance) 31, 35, 55, 99
Alrutz, M. 105
applied theatre in paediatrics 97–101; actions by artists to improve 111–112; actions by healthcare providers to improve 110–111; actions by local authorities and governments to improve 111; act of caring and 15–16; anxiety in hospitals and 62–63; defined 98; dramatic frame in 63–64; eudaimonia and 4–6; fictional bubble in 14–15, 50; future of 108–113; marginal participant technique in 16–18; participatory activities incorporated into 5; play therapy *versus* 11–14; reflective poetry and 78–84; as research 2, 66–68; sick children's stories in (*see* sick children's stories); as synergistic and eudemonic phenomenon 1–6; theatrical space in hospitals and 8–9
Aristotle 4, 12
artists: emotions of 78–91, self-care of 78, 85–86, 90; training of 78–94; wellbeing of 79, 86, 87, 89–91, 94
arts-based interventions 98, 105, 107
arts and health: definition of 4, 11; development of 97, 109–110, 111
Atkinson, P. 16
attunement 9–11
audiences 14–15

audience participation 1, 3, 12, 16–18, 32, 58, 92, 99
audience evaluation: interviews in 62
authority 98, 111
awareness, emotional 87–90

bedside theatre: 3, 4, 21; bedside entertainment 34; bedside methodology 23–28
bereaved children 39–41
Bird Island project 60–61; 'Lollie the rough collie and the magic kiss' story 61, 120–122; puppetry in 64–66
Boal, A. 6, 12, 56
Bolton, G. 69
Bourke, J. 55
Boyd, B. 105
Brodzinski, E. 12
burn victims 33–35

Carel, H. H. 54
care 15–16, 29, 52, 58, 65, 78–79, 83–84, 113
caring, act of 15–16; for the artists 85–87; emotional awareness as 87–90
Carter, B. 68
child healthcare 17, 32, 58, 60, 111–112
child stress 5, 13, 16, 22, 84–85; applied performance addressing 62–63, 69, 72, 75; sick children's stories of 53, 55–56
children as patients 3, 10, 21, 56–58, 70, 88–89, 99

clinical stressors 11, 53, 55, 75, 102
children: bereaved 39–41; as burn victims 33–35; communicating pain and fear 9–11, 68–72; in critical care 43–45; in denial 45–46; as dialysis patients 46–47; feeling anxiety in hospitals 62–63; locked-in syndrome in 72–73; with long-life conditions 37–39; as long-term patients 46–47; meaning of images and words in stories of 7–8; as oncology patients 47–49; research on hospitalised 66–68; stories of sick (*see* sick children's stories); surgery in 35–37; transitioning from home to hospital 66; as transplant patients 74–75; with visual impairment 42–43
communication between child and artist 55
communication between child and parent 57–58, 71
communication between child and nurse 53, 74
community engagement 79, 90–92, 107–108
compassion 4, 5, 16, 62, 72, 88–92; in care 84–85; sick children's stories and 32, 33, 54–57
Conlon, C. 102
COVID-19 pandemic 13, 18, 21, 25, 97; impact on Rocket-Arts 29–30; recommendations for learning post- 101–108
creativity 3, 4, 7, 10, 21, 34, 37, 66, 98, 100, 105
critical care, children in 43–45

Danton, L. 39
denial, children in 45–46
de Saint-Exupéry, A. 4
dialysis patients 46–47
digital performance: digital film 26, 29, 103; digital storytelling 25–30, 103–106
disability 27, 103
dramatherapy 32–33, 53, 55, 63–64, 69
dramatic frame 63–64
Dramaturgical Model of social interaction 10–11

Edmiston, B. 63
education 5, 12, 32, 66, 71, 107, 109–110; actor training 79–94; health education 58, 60, 67
embodied experience/knowledge 79
emotional awareness 87–90
emotional regulation 90–92
emotional resilience 89–90

emotional safety 89
emotional skills in artists 78; caring for the artist and 85–87; emotional awareness as act of caring and 87–90; emotional intelligence 86, 88; emotional regulation and 90–92; portrait of excellent 92–94; reflective poetry in paediatrics and 78–84; training in 90–92; as walking the labyrinth on the ward 84–85
empathy 10, 88–89
empowerment 14, 45, 56
ethics 2–3, 7, 13, 16–17, 27, 68, 78, 98, 101, 106, 112; actors and 90, 92; sick children's stories and 29, 33, 54, 58
eudaimonia 4–6
excellent actor, portrait of 92–94
expression of pain 10, 68
evaluation of the arts and arts in health 1, 31, 67; challenges 78, 85, 101, 103; cost-effectiveness 107, 111

fictional bubble 14–15, 50
film 21, 25–26, 29, 52, 98, 103, 106
Fisher, A. 90
Fitzpatrick, T. 25
Fourie, A. 66
fuzzy boundaries 2–3
funding 107, 108, 111

Gallagher, M. W. 4
Goffman, E. 10–11
Goleman, D. 88, 91
Gottschall, J. 7

Hägg-Martinell, A. 17–18
Hammersley, M. 16
Hänninen, V. 11
Hepplewhite, V. 10
health 5, 17; healthcare professionals 9, 15, 28, 36, 57–58, 65, 86, 91, 98, 104, 106–111; training 93–94, 107
healthcare projects: arts in 16, 57–58, 67, 102
Hopkinson, C. 79
hospitals: feeling worried in 62–63; labyrinth metaphor in 84–85; locked-in syndrome in 72–73; theatrical space in 8–9
hospital performance 55, 87
hospital space 17, 46, 51, 53
hospital theatre 7
Howell, C. 2

identity of illness 24, 31, 55
imagery 85

imagination 2, 6, 10, 11, 13, 14, 22, 26, 28, 32, 36, 41, 45, 84, 98, 100; co-imagination 105; emotional-revealing elements in 54; enabling metaxis 7–8; hospitals existing in 63; puppetry and 61, 66, 67, 71
improvisation 21, 23, 24, 29, 32, 51, 88, 94, 100, 107
Illingworth, S. 79

Jack, K. 79

Kamei-Hannan, C. 42
Karypidou, A. 79, 85–86, 88
Koinis, A. 86
Kourtidou-Sextou, E. 85

labyrinth metaphor in hospital setting 84–85
Lascaratou, C. 9, 41, 48, 53, 68
Lee, K. J. 91
Leino-Kilpi, H. 9
Lerwick, J. 10, 62
limited-English speakers 73–74
'Little Prince, The' 4
locked-in syndrome 72–73
'Lollie the rough collie and the magic kiss' story 61, 120–122
long-life conditions, children with 37–39
long-term patients 46–47

marginal participant technique 16–18
Mayer, J. D. 91
McCormick, E. 57, 85
medication 5, 13, 37, 51, 56, 113
mental health 10, 62
metaphor 2, 6–7, 8, 10–11, 14, 32, 36, 52, 63, 79, 84–85, 98, 99; illness and 41, 48–49
methodology: diaries 28, 68; mixed 62; qualitative 67–68; quantitative 68; video 34, 39
mindfulness 10, 24, 55, 89, 94, 101
metaxis 6–7, 15, 52
'Moon made of cheese, A' (Sheila) 35–37
Moss, H. 85
'My grandfather's wellies' (Alex) 39–42

'Naughty wolf, The' (Paul) 37–39
NHS (national health service) 21, 23, 25, 58, 60
'No!' (Karim) 45–46
not knowing, experience of 4
nurses 15, 45–46, 50, 53, 62, 71, 79, 84, 109; nursing practice 79

oncology patients 47–49
O'Neill, D. 85
O'Toole, J. 6, 7, 63
Oyebode, F. 83–84
ownership of the performance 2–3, 5, 29, 37, 50, 62, 80, 91, 93

pain and fear, communicating 9–11, 68–72
'Park for the animals, A' (Margaret) 49–52
participation and interaction 1–4, 15, 43–44, 55, 58, 64, 68, 100; audience 32, 92, 99; marginal 16–18
participatory arts-based activities 5, 12
participatory theatre 12, 14, 57, 69, 71, 108–109; performance 2–3
partnership 98, 106, 108–109, 110, 111
Pascal, B. 4
Pelander, T. 9
'Piano is on fire, The' (Jane) 33–35
'Planetary, The' (Melissa) 47–49
play, therapeutic 11–14
poetry, reflective 78–84
policy(ies) about the arts and health 102, 107, 108
post-pandemic learning recommendations 101–108
practice as research 32
Preston, S. 79
puppetry: dramatic frame and 63–64; participatory, in hospital 64–66
public health 25, 102

qualitative research 67–68

reflective poetry 78–84
regulation, emotional 90–92
relaxation (in performance) 37, 65, 72, 103
research evaluation 16, 111
resilience 89–90
'Robot who could not dance, A' (Lisa) 46–47
Rocket-Arts project 21–30, 90, 103–105; collection of stories in 26–28; impact of COVID-19 on 29–30; post-pandemic digital solutions in 25–26; pre-pandemic bedside performance in 23–25; script for 115–119; sick children's stories in (see sick children's stories); story in 22

safety, emotional 89
Sakr, Y. 3
Salovey, P. 91
Scarry, E. 53
school teachers as research participants 67
Sepinuck, T. 3–4, 11
Sextou, P. 79, 85–86, 88

sick children's stories 31; Alex: 'My grandfather's wellies' 39–42; Claire: 'Silence' 43–45; of hospitalisation on a stitched land 52–58; introduction to 31–33; Jane: 'The piano is on fire' 33–35; Karim: 'No!' 45–46; Lisa: 'A robot who could not dance' 46–47; Margaret: 'A park for the animals' 49–52; Melissa: 'The Planetary' 47–49; Paul: 'The naughty wolf' 37–39; Sandy: 'We need the pancakes' 42–43; Sheila: 'A moon made of cheese' 35–37
'Silence' (Claire) 43–45
Simons, J. 68
Singh, S. 102
site-specific performance 8, 99
Smith, M. 66
Socratic method 17
Stanford, E. A. 9
Steinke, S. 67
stitched land, stories of hospitalisation on 52–58
stories: co-creation with vulnerable people 3; fictional bubble in 14–15, 50; of hospitalisation on stitched land 52–58; in-betweenness of 6–9; meaning of images and words in children's 7–8; metaxis and 6–7, 15, 52; Rocket-Arts 26–28; of sick children (*see* sick children's stories); synergies of 3–4; understanding pain through 9–11
storytelling 5, 7–8, 12; digital 21, 23, 26; puppetry 65, 71; sick children's stories 31, 34–37, 41, 42–43, 51, 54, 56–57
stress and anxiety 44, 61, 68, 72, 85, 87, 102; over hospitalisation 62; perioperative 12; pre-operative 16, 22, 35–37, 55; separation 40
symbolism 31, 40, 42, 84, 89
synergy 1–2, 33, 36, 49, 72, 93, 98, 100–101
synergistic performance 2, 13, 25, 33, 90, 100, 104
synergistic relationship 92
surgery in children 35–37
sympathy 10
synergy 1–2

Theatre of the Oppressed 56
Theatre of Witness 3–4
Thompson, J. 29, 90
transformation 8–9, 13–14, 28, 66
transplant patients 74–75
trauma and traumatic experience 12–13, 34, 53, 65, 75, 79, 99

visual impairment 42–43

wellbeing (children) 4–5, 11–13, 32, 86, 98, 101, 102; digital arts-based interventions for 62; emotional awareness and 87–90, 91, 94; reflective practice and 79; theatre as vehicle of transformation of 13–16
wellbeing (social) 5, 13, 86, 102
wellbeing (self-care) 78, 86
wellbeing, eudemonic 4
'We need the pancakes' (Sandy) 42–43
Winston's Wish 41

Yang, Y. 35